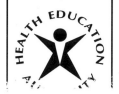

Improving Infant Health

The effectiveness of health promotion activities to reduce still birth, infant mortality and morbidity: a literature review

Jo Garcia
Merry France-Dawson
Alison Macfarlane

National Perinatal Epidemiology Unit, Oxford

© Crown Copyright Reserved 1994

Published by
Health Education Authority
Hamilton House
Mabledon Place
London WC1H 9TX.

ISBN 0 7521 0230 3

Typeset by BookEns Ltd, Baldock, Herts.
Printed in Great Britain

Contents

Acknowledgements

This review was commissioned and funded by the Health Education Authority and carried out by Jo Garcia, Merry France-Dawson and Alison Macfarlane of the National Perinatal Epidemiology Unit, Oxford, which is funded by the Department of Health. Opinions expressed in this report are those of the researchers alone and do not necessarily reflect the views of the Department of Health. The HEA project team responsible for this report was Isobel Bowler, Karen Ford and Andrea Young (now at North Thames Region). We would like to thank colleagues at the Maternity Alliance, the Toxoplasmosis Trust and the National Childbirth Trust. Thanks are also due to Josephine Green at the Centre for Family Research, Cambridge University; Monique Kaminski of INSERM in Paris; and Ann Johnson, Natalie Kenney and other colleagues at the National Perinatal Epidemiology Unit. Jane Thomas of London University and Mary Renfrew of NPEU made important contributions to the sections on diet in pregnancy and breastfeeding respectively.

The report benefited from the comments of the following internal and external reviewers: Colleagues at the Department of Health; Jean Chapple, North West Thames RHA; Michael Corr, HEA; Adam Crosier, HEA; Kathy Elliott, HEA; Melanie Every, Royal College of Midwives Trust; Shirley Goodwin, Health Services Consultant; Chris Gowdridge, Maternity Alliance; Mary Sayers, HEA; Lynn Stockley, HEA; Rae Magowan, Trent RHA; Caroline Woodroffe, London University Institute of Child Health; Hilary Whent, HEA.

Foreword

The reduction of still birth, infant mortality and morbidity offers great opportunities for health gain. In England still birth and infant mortality rates have fallen considerably in the last 20 years, but there is still scope for improvement. *The Health of the Nation: A strategy for health in England* stresses the importance of sustaining and building upon this progress in improving children's health outcomes, and the NHS has been called upon to shift its focus towards disease prevention and health promotion. At local level, purchasing for health gain requires a good knowledge base, including information on the effectiveness of different health-related interventions.

The Health Education Authority, as the national agency for health education and as part of the NHS, aims to help others in the health service to develop local health strategies. This review follows on from the 1993 report *Reducing Childhood Accidents*, and has been commissioned as part of HEA work on child health. It is intended to inform purchasers on what might be included in a list of 'best buys' in health promotion.

Although there is a great deal of health promotion aimed at improving infant health outcomes, there is relatively little rigorous evaluation of these activities. Nevertheless, there are some randomised controlled trials, and it is possible and worthwhile to assess and grade the evidence from many of the less rigorous evaluations.

This literature review is intended primarily for those who are deciding where to invest scarce resources, but it may also be useful to those health professionals who work with pregnant women and young families. We hope that in bringing together all the evidence in this wide area it will contribute to local and national policy development.

Isobel Bowler
Karen Ford
HEA, 1994

Summary

In England still birth and infant mortality rates have fallen considerably in the last 20 years. In 1992, the stillbirth rate was 4.2 per 1000 live births, compared with 12.9 in 1970. For neonatal mortality the rate was 4.3 deaths per 1000 live births in 1992, compared with 12.3 in 1970. In contrast, the post-neonatal mortality rate fell very little from the mid 1970s onwards, until it fell from 4.1 per 1000 live births in 1988 to 2.3 in 1992.

This review is an evaluation of research into health promotion activities aimed at reducing the rates of still birth, infant mortality, ill-health and disability in childhood. Other important social and emotional outcomes of health promotion have not been covered explicitly. The overall aim of the review is to provide information on the most effective forms of intervention. We therefore need to ask three questions. First, what are the likely areas for health promotion interventions? In other words, has epidemiological research identified associations between poor outcomes and particular aspects of behaviour or lifestyle? Second, what is the evidence that health promotion interventions affect the relevant behaviour or lifestyle factors? Third, what is the evidence that health promotion interventions improve health outcomes for babies? It is hoped that this will prove useful to policy makers, purchasers, commissioners, managers and practitioners in the planning and development of work for health promotion.

The review covers research published between 1985 and 1993, both national and international. Published reports of research on interventions that aim to promote infant and child health and reduce mortality were identified through bibliographic searches using the Cochrane Collaboration Pregnancy and Childbirth Module (CCPC), formerly the Oxford Database of Perinatal Trials (ODPT), Medline Database, Index Medicus and the On Line Minicom System at the Health Education Authority.

The research that we have reviewed makes it clear that there is potential for using health promotion to improve health outcomes for babies, although inevitably some aspects are more likely to respond to changes in health care and wider social and political actions. So far, though, few studies of health promotion interventions have shown reliably that reductions in mortality or major morbidity can be achieved. The recent striking fall in the rate of cot deaths may prove to be an exception to this. Further primary research is needed; in some areas, such as smoking, there is a core of evaluative research to build on; in others, such as the prevention of neural tube defects, clinical research has shown the benefits that can be achieved, and this needs to be followed by evaluations of health promotion directed to users and care-givers. As new research about effective clinical and other interventions becomes available, new topics for health promotion will certainly emerge. Specific conclusions that arise from the review are drawn together here. Recommendations for research are at the end of the report.

Key findings

- Behavioural self-help strategies seem to be the most effective way of helping women to stop smoking during pregnancy.

- Small reductions in smoking could be obtained by advice only.

- Interventions aimed at reducing smoking can lead to small increases in average birthweight, but so far have not been shown to reduce perinatal mortality, preterm delivery or the proportion of low-birthweight babies.

- Interventions aimed at reducing consumption of alcohol should be targeted at heavy drinkers, partly because of the low levels of self-reported consumption among pregnant women.

- Health promotion advice in pregnancy should reinforce the general messages about personal and food hygiene and thorough cooking which are important for all the UK population in the light of the increasing levels of illness due to foodborne pathogens.

- On the basis of currently available evidence it appears that for the well nourished majority of women changes to diet are unlikely to result in significant changes in pregnancy outcomes. Health promotion for these mothers should emphasise the messages of a varied and adequate diet following current 'healthy eating' guidelines. Vitamin D and folic acid are the only nutrients for which supplementation should routinely be advised for all pregnant women.

- General health promotion for adolescents should include activities designed to discourage inappropriate slimming, so that those who become pregnant are less likely to have low prepregnancy weights and depleted nutritional reserves. Health promotion in pregnancy for this group, particularly younger adolescents, should emphasise the importance of iron, calcium and folic acid in the diet.

- It is possible that more significant benefits may be achieved by an improvement in the diets of women from low income groups. Within the context of advice for all mothers particular emphasis should be placed on promoting the consumption of adequate amounts of food with increased nutrient density.

- There is probably a continuing need to emphasise the importance of Vitamin D intake, as well as vitamin B_{12} and folate in health promotion designed for women of Asian descent.

- The benefits of increasing intake of folate around the time of conception have been demonstrated experimentally, but there is an urgent need for research into the design of effective strategies for the public and health professionals to change behaviour.

- There appears to be no evidence that justifies or rejects any form of dietary intervention specifically aimed at preventing pre-eclampsia during pregnancy.

- It is difficult to interpret studies on the effect of paid work on pregnant women as women doing physically hard or unpleasant work often have other poor circumstances which confound the results of studies.

- A recent review of the relevant randomised controlled trials found that there was not enough evidence to draw conclusions about the effects (both positive and negative) of vigorous recreational exercise on pregnancy outcomes. Data available indicate that moderate aerobic activity is safe and beneficial for most women.

- Education programmes that highlight the risk to the fetus of poor pet, personal and food hygiene are acceptable to pregnant women and can have a positive effect on hygiene behaviours, thereby potentially reducing the incidence of congenital toxoplasmosis.

- Apart from steps to improve the accessibility and quality of care, and to encourage general practitioners to refer some women promptly, there are unlikely to be significant health gains in untargeted health promotion aimed at bringing all pregnant women in for care earlier. However, this is unlikely to be true for particular subgroups of women, for whom early antenatal advice and care can improve outcomes.

- Specific health-promotion campaigns, such as the Asian Mother and Baby Campaign and the Hackney advocacy project, have had some success at improving access to health information and health care more appropriate to their needs for some minority ethnic groups.

- Women having antenatal care are generally underinformed about the tests they are being offered and which they may subsequently undergo. If women are to be active participants in decision making about what antenatal tests to undergo, they must be provided with adequate information. This should include the purpose of testing, the condition(s) being screened for, the likelihood that an abnormality will be detected, the test procedures, any risks involved, the meaning of positive and negative test results, and possible actions for a positive result. These include termination, preparing for the birth of a handicapped child and adoption.

- Improving knowledge without creating positive attitudes about breastfeeding does not increase the incidence or duration of breastfeeding. Knowledge on its own seems to be less important than socially acquired attitudes in influencing women to breastfeed.

- The use of lactation counsellors appears to have enhanced women's abilities to maintain breastfeeding for as long as they want to, particularly in women from lower socioeconomic groups. Encouragement and support in problem solving was more effective than early initiation of feeding, increased frequency of feeds and discouraging of supplementary feeds.

- The provision of artificial milk in discharge packs may pose a risk to the duration of breastfeeding. Providing a breast pump, but no artificial milk, in discharge packs is seen to increase the duration of breastfeeding.

- Women who fed their babies within two hours after birth, and who fed their babies when they needed, continued to breastfeed for longer and had fewer problems than women who delayed the first feed for four hours and who fed on a fixed schedule.

- Women who experience painful nipples when breastfeeding are more likely to continue to breastfeed if they are taught to reposition the baby at the breast so that feeding does not hurt.

- Evaluations of infant car restraint loan schemes show modest benefits in terms of correct use.

Note

At the start of each risk factor section the following information is given:

Potential impact of health promotion at population level This is the potential for health-promotion activities aimed at a particular risk behaviour to produce health gain at a population level.

Potential impact of health promotion on individuals This the potential for health-promotion activities aimed at particular risk behaviour to have an effect on infant health outcomes at an individual level, even if at a population level the improvement will be minimal because of the rarity of the risk behaviour.

Relevant research This gives an indication of the quality of research in the area.

Evidence of impact on behaviour This indicates whether there are rigorous studies that identify the health-promotion interventions which can alter the risk behaviour.

Evidence of impact on outcomes This indicates whether there are studies which have linked the intervention, via behaviour change, to an improvement in infant health outcomes. NB: this is very rare; a 'no' in this section does not mean that health promotion does not affect outcomes, only that there have been no studies that have demonstrated this.

Section
1
Introduction

'The promotion of maternal and infant health should begin before conception and continue throughout pregnancy and delivery and beyond, into infancy'.[1]

This statement, made by the Department of Health in 1990, reflects the emphasis given to health-promotion interventions concerned with the health of women and babies. In the strategy for health in England, *The Health of the Nation*, the Department expressed the view that the goal for women's and children's health must be 'sustaining and building on progress which has already been made'.[2]

There are numerous influences that affect unborn babies and their chances of surviving the pregnancy, birth and the first year of life. Being born too soon, too small, ill or in adverse social or economic circumstances can pose risks to the life of the young child.[3-5] Where these do not result in death, babies who survive may have chronic health problems or disabilities.

Although many of these risks are clearly influenced by particular practices and environments, others are less amenable to change by individuals and those who offer care to them. Health-promotion interventions in pregnancy are aimed at encouraging and supporting parents to adopt and sustain healthy life practices, thereby reducing risk factors believed to be harmful to the good health of the family.[6] They are also designed to encourage prospective parents to use the health services available to them and to take their own decisions, both individually and collectively, to improve their health status and environment.

The main part of this review examines research on the effectiveness of health-promotion strategies which aim to reduce ill-health in newborn babies. Factors that can adversely affect the unborn baby will be discussed and interventions to reduce them evaluated. The review also evaluates research into interventions aimed at promoting the health of babies during the first year of life.

1.1 Aims of the review

This review is an evaluation of research into health-promotion activities intended to reduce the rates of still birth, infant mortality, ill-health and disability in childhood. The overall aim is to provide information on the most effective forms of intervention. We therefore need to ask three questions. First, what are the likely areas for health-promotion interventions? In other words, has epidemiological research identified associations between poor outcomes and particular aspects of behaviour or lifestyle? Second, what is the evidence that health-promotion interventions affect the relevant behaviour or lifestyle factors? Third, what is the evidence that health-promotion interventions improve health outcomes for babies? An example is presented to illustrate this.

Diet in pregnancy – a complex story

There is evidence that some pregnant women eat diets that would be considered inadequate for any adult woman, and that thin women and those with poor weight gain in pregnancy are more likely to have babies of low birthweight.

Offering women balanced food supplements in pregnancy leads to a small improvement in the mothers' average weight gain, mean birthweight, birth length and head circumference. Where babies have been followed up, however, there has not been any indication so far of better growth or health in infancy. A potential risk of dietary supplementation, particularly where women have been very poorly nourished, is that improved fetal growth will lead to increased complications at delivery, but this has not been investigated so far. In addition, some women who gain a lot of weight in pregnancy may find it hard to return to an appropriate weight after birth. Giving women advice about diet, as opposed to prescribing supplements, has also been shown to lead to changes in eating habits, and in one study to small improvements in birthweight.

Until we have some evidence about the longer-term balance of risks and benefits, for mother and infant, of changes to diet in pregnancy, health promotion about diet should be seen as of general benefit to the mother's health rather than a method of improving pregnancy outcome.

One exception to this is likely to be advice about folate around the time of conception. The detailed evidence is still incomplete, but trials show that supplementation with folate reduces the recurrence of neural tube defects and, with multivitamins, reduces the first occurrence of such defects. Further work is needed to evaluate health-promotion interventions aimed at encouraging improved diets or the use of dietary supplements, since women are not usually in contact with the health services around the time of conception.

In addition, the advice given to adolescent girls and other vulnerable groups may be particularly important, but further research is crucial to identify effective means of improving their diet and monitoring outcome.

1.2 Still birth and infant mortality

In 1980 the House of Commons Social Services Committee's *Report on Perinatal and Neonatal Mortality*, usually known as the Short Report,[7] suggested that 'factors causing perinatal and neonatal mortality and handicap broadly divide into two categories'. The first category was made up of medical factors which may or may not be preventable. The Committee included both lack of health care on the one hand and congenital malformations incompatible with life on the other. This leaves aside the question of the effectiveness of specific aspects of care in preventing mortality. The second category, described as generally preventable, was made up of socioeconomic and other factors 'such as lack of education, poverty, poor housing, possibly poor nutrition, unplanned pregnancy, smoking, drinking alcohol to excess, etc.'[7] There are a large number of factors which may affect both mortality rates and the health of babies. Reducing social disadvantage would therefore have an impact on perinatal mortality and morbidity. However, its effects are likely to take place in the longer rather than the shorter term, and this review focuses on shorter-term strategies concerned with lifestyle and the use of health care.

Table 1 Still births and infant mortality rates per 1000 live, and live and still births, England

Year	Still-birth rate	Perinatal mortality rate	Neonatal mortality rate	Post-neonatal mortality rate	Infant mortality rate
1960	19.5	32.5	15.3	6.3	21.6
1970	12.9	23.4	12.3	5.9	18.2
1980	7.3	13.4	7.6	4.4	12.0
1990	4.6	8.1	4.6	3.3	7.9
1992	4.2	7.6	4.3	2.3	6.5

Still-birth rate: Late fetal deaths after 28 weeks' gestation, per 1000 total births. On 1 October 1992 the limit was lowered to 24 weeks, but still-births at 24–27 weeks registered in the last quarter of 1992 have been omitted for consistency.

Perinatal
mortality rate: Still births and deaths in the first week of life, per 1000 total births.

Neonatal
mortality rate: Deaths at less than 28 days of life, per 1000 live births.

Post-neonatal
mortality rate: Deaths at ages 28 days and over and under 1 year, per 1000 live births.

Infant mortality: Deaths aged under 1, per 1000 live births.

Still birth and infant mortality rates have fallen considerably over the past 20 years or so. The still birth rate for England was 4.2 in 1992, compared with 12.9 in 1970.[8] (For consistency, the rate for 1992 omits the still births born at 24–27 weeks' gestation after the criteria for registration was lowered to 24 weeks on 1 October, 1992.) The fall was particularly dramatic between the mid

1970s and mid 1980s, as Figure 1 shows. This period also shows a similar decrease in neonatal mortality, shown in Figure 2. The rate was 4.3 deaths per 1000 live births in 1992, compared with 12.3 in 1970. In contrast, post-neonatal mortality rates declined very little from the mid 1970s onwards, until they fell from 4.1 per 1000 live births in 1988 to 2.3 in 1992.[8] Thus although the decline in mortality was considerable overall, there were marked differences between the pattern shown by still birth, neonatal mortality and perinatal mortality rates on the one hand, and post-neonatal mortality rates on the other. The differences can also be seen geographically and between groups within the population.[8,9]

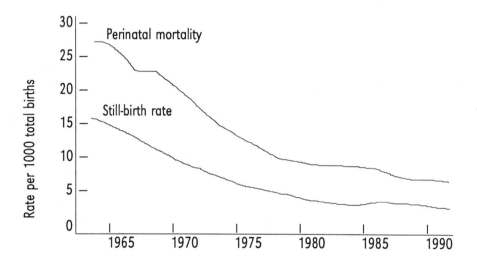

Figure 1   Perinatal mortality and still-birth rates, England and Wales, 1965–92
Source: OPCS Mortality statistics. Series DH3

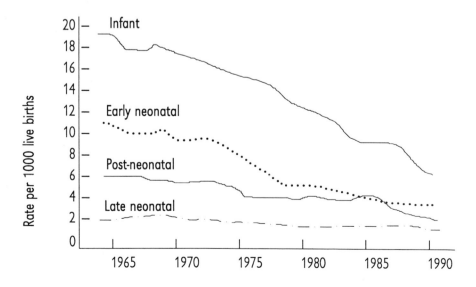

Figure 2   Deaths in the first year of life, England and Wales, 1965–92

Source: OPCS Mortality statistics. Series DH3

Over the past 20 years perinatal mortality rates have fallen in all NHS regions, but the relative differences between the highest and the lowest rates have remained. In most years, the rates for the West Midlands region is about one and a half times that of the East Anglian region. In contrast, differences in post-neonatal mortality narrowed rapidly in the early 1970s and regional differences have been relatively small ever since.

Similar patterns can be seen when mortality rates are tabulated by the socioeconomic group of the baby's father. Although perinatal mortality rates have fallen in all manual and non manual groups, the differentials have been maintained. In contrast, post-neonatal mortality rates for babies with fathers in manual occupations fell throughout the 1970s and began to level off in the 1980s, before falling in 1991. Among babies with fathers in non-manual occupations, post-neonatal mortality rates levelled off during the 1970s. Thus although there are still marked socioeconomic differences in post-neonatal mortality, these are narrower than they were in 1970–72.[8] Unfortunately, these tabulations are restricted to babies born within marriage. A special analysis for the House of Commons Health Committee gave a more detailed breakdown of births outside marriage than usually appears in published tables.[10] This showed that neonatal and post-neonatal mortality rates were higher for births outside marriage than within marriage, and that post-neonatal mortality rates were higher for mothers registering the births on their own. Of births within marriage, and those registered outside marriage by both parents, mortality was highest when the father recorded no paid employment.

Mortality is not tabulated by ethnic group because parents' ethnic origin is not recorded at birth registration.[9,11] It would require legislation to change this. Country of birth is an increasingly poor proxy for both 'race' and 'ethnicity'. Those who are not 'ethnically' white British but were born in Britain – the increasing number of second- and third-generation black and Asian people, Irish, Jewish or traveller people – are missed. The majority of African-Caribbean women now of childbearing age were born in the UK to parents who migrated in the 1950s and 1960s. More recently, Asian women born in the UK have begun to enter the childbearing age range.

When mortality rates are tabulated by the mother's country of birth, babies of women born in Pakistan stand out as having high still birth and infant mortality rates, whereas those for babies born to women from elsewhere are not much higher than those for women born in the UK.[8] Babies born to Pakistani women have a comparatively high incidence of congenital malformations.[12–15]

Still birth and infant mortality rates are particularly high among babies born too soon or too small.[8] Although there is some difference between the causes and problems associated with being born before term and those of being born at term but too small, these cannot be monitored in national statistics as gestational age is not recorded when registering live births in England and Wales.

The very smallest babies have mortality rates which are high but which have fallen rapidly in recent years, giving rise to concern about the quality of life of survivors.[3] The prevention of preterm birth is therefore a major objective of health professionals and parents. Being born later, but small for dates, is more difficult to detect in advance and the scope for prevention is less clear. As Figure 3 shows, low birthweight is more common among babies with fathers in manual occupations than among those in non-manual occupations.[8]

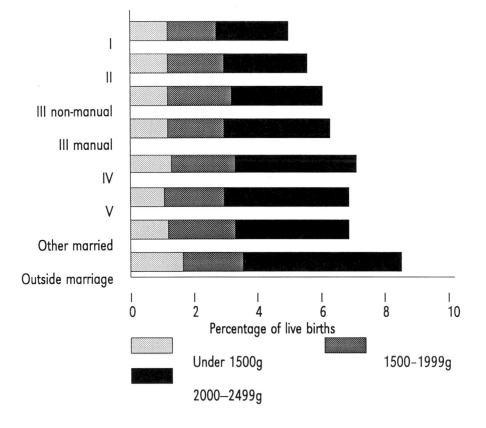

Figure 3 Low birthweight by father's socioeconomic group, England and Wales, 1990
Source: OPCS mortality statistics Series DH3

Factors associated with low birthweight are numerous, and are confounded with each other. They include maternal age, education, height and prepregnancy weight, family income, parity, birth interval,[16-18] physical effort, isolation, living conditions, lack of social support,[19-21] inadequate access to and uptake of services and information,[4] maternal emotional crises, unplanned pregnancy,[5] previous low birthweight,[22] smoking during pregnancy, diet and alcohol use during pregnancy.[16]

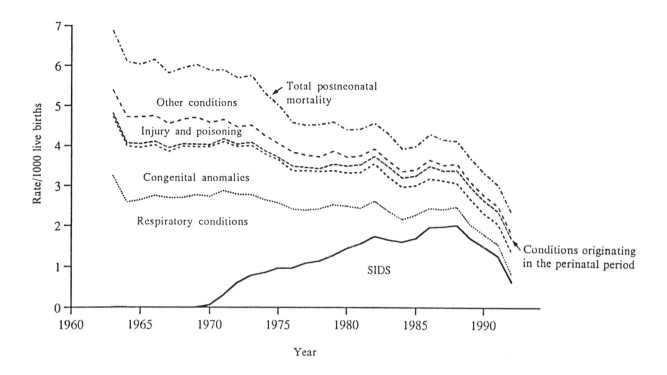

Figure 4 Cumulative postneonatal mortality rates by certified cause of death, England and Wales, 1963–1992
Source: OPCS mortality statistics, series DH3.

The decrease in deaths attributed to the sudden infant death syndrome or to respiratory disease made a major contribution to the rapid decline in post-neonatal mortality from 1989 onwards, shown in Figure 4. The fall in numbers of deaths with 'sudden infant death' as their underlying cause accounted for over three-quarters of the fall in the overall rate between 1988 and 1992.[23] In 1990, 'sudden infant death' accounted for 45 per cent of post-neonatal deaths and the rate was 39 per cent higher for boys than for girls. Congenital anomalies made up 15 per cent of post-neonatal deaths for boys and 17 per cent for girls. Injury and poisoning accounted for only 4 per cent of deaths for boys and 3 per cent for girls, and the rate of death for these causes in both sexes has nearly halved since 1980.

Socioeconomic differences in post-neonatal mortality are considerable. For births within marriage, the rate varied from 1.8 per 1000 for babies with fathers in professional occupations to 3.7 per 1000 for those in unskilled manual occupations.

1.3 Illness and disability in babies

Health in childhood is also affected by a variety of factors, including parents' unemployment, low income, socioeconomic group, unfavourable environments and lifestyle.[3, 4, 24] Some children may be born with specific genetic conditions such as cystic fibrosis and Tay–Sachs disease,[24] sickle-cell conditions and thalassaemia.[25,26] Sickle-cell and thalassaemia are generally believed to be restricted to certain ethnic groups, which is incorrect, although they are more common among African, Caribbean, Asian, Arab and southern European people than others such as northern Europeans.[25,26] In the same way, cystic fibrosis is more common among white northern Europeans. Screening during pregnancy can identify pregnancies 'at risk' for some genetic conditions. In addition to these specific conditions, low-birthweight babies who survive are more likely than larger babies to have major disabilities. They are also more likely to be smaller and have more neurological problems than children whose birthweights were average.[3]

1.4   Scope for intervention

Some factors that lead to infant death and poor health outcomes are not readily amenable to health-promotion interventions, or even health-service interventions. Health promotion is used to attempt to minimise some obvious risk factors and thereby increase the possibility of positive outcomes. It can also be directed to improving the uptake of care – ideally, care that is known to be effective. Although it may be shown that individual risk factors contribute to intrauterine growth retardation and preterm birth, the full extent of that contribution is not always clearly measurable because of confounding with other risk factors. It is difficult, therefore to assess the extent to which the factors are themselves causal and to measure the extent to which they are confounded with other factors which may be causal. Thus, it is difficult to estimate in advance the precise effect of health-promotion interventions. Nevertheless, randomised controlled trials can look for effects of particular health-promotion interventions on the relevant behaviours and on the outcomes in question, because they can set up groups that differ only in respect of the intervention being tested.

1.5   Health promotion activities

Health promotion has been defined as 'any planned measure which promotes health or prevents disease, disability and premature death'.[27] It therefore encompasses health education and much more. Healthy public policy and health education work together as part of the process of health promotion.[27]

Because more women use antenatal care than antenatal classes, it has been suggested that this should be main setting for health promotion.[28] At present, the antenatal clinic is generally the first point of call at the hospital for pregnant women, usually at about 10–12 weeks' gestation, after the pregnancy has been confirmed by their general practitioner (GP). The implementation of the Expert Maternity Group's recommendations in *Changing Childbirth*[29] means that this is likely to change in the future, with more antenatal care, including booking, taking place in the community, and an increase in the extent to which midwives are the lead professionals. When GPs and midwives see women early in their pregnancies they have an important opportunity for health promotion that they may not be using fully at present.[28] 'Lay' contributions to health-promotion activities come from many voluntary and maternity organisations, such as the Maternity Alliance, the National Childbirth Trust and the Child Accident Prevention Trust.

Routine antenatal care involves a large number of health professionals, including midwives, GPs, obstetricians, physiotherapists, health visitors and paediatricians. Some of these also make a large contribution to postnatal care and promoting the health of babies in the community.[29] Antenatal care focuses on the health of the mother and the developing fetus. This is monitored during pregnancy, and screening and diagnostic tests are carried out to look for abnormalities.

In addition to antenatal care, it is usual to provide antenatal classes. Some are for women only, others welcome partners or friends and yet others are for specific groups such as diabetic women and women whose first language is not English. The numbers of classes available differ greatly from place to place, and classes may be run by the hospital, local midwives or health visitors, local GPs or health centres.[30] Antenatal classes, generally offered in the third trimester, usually consist of six to eight meetings and are designed to examine and discuss issues such as health during pregnancy, labour and parenting skills. After the birth, postnatal classes and child health clinics, combined with a system for recalling babies for periodic check-ups, provide some continuity of care for mothers and their babies.[28,29]

A large number of publications are produced by both statutory and voluntary organisations, and many are distributed free to women. These include the HEA's *The Pregnancy Book,*[31], and others produced by midwives and obstetricians, such as the 'Bounty' books.[32,33] All of these publications stress the importance of antenatal care and attending antenatal classes. Other publications are designed to help mothers cope with their new babies and the problems that may occur. These include publications by the HEA, such as *Birth to Five*, and a variety of leaflets on immunisation, breastfeeding, weaning and maternal and child health clinics,[34-38] some of which are translated into languages other than English. Yet other leaflets about the practical and financial aspects of pregnancy and baby care are produced by maternity and voluntary organisations, trades unions and companies.[39-43]

Overall, extensive local and national resources are put into the whole range of health-promotion activities for childbearing women and their families. There is clearly a need for information about the value of these activities to be assembled and made widely available. This should help to guide those who purchase and provide services, and also highlight areas where research is needed.

1.6 Methods of the review

Published reports of research on interventions which aim to promote the health of mothers and babies and reduce mortality were identified through bibliographic searches. The databases used were the Oxford Database of Perinatal Trials (ODPT) (now called the Cochrane Collaboration Pregnancy and Childbirth Module), Medline Database, Index Medicus and the On Line Minicom System at the Health Education Authority.

This review covers research published in English between 1985 and 1993, both in the UK and internationally. Definitive work which has made a major contribution to the literature has been included regardless of when it was published. Peer-reviewed articles and clinical trials, conference abstracts and unpublished work have also been used. The majority of this material is focused on the antenatal period and the first year of life.

1.7 Coverage of the review

Our brief was to focus on health-promotion interventions that take place during the childbearing period and which are likely to affect mortality and health in the first year of life. In order to fulfil this and to keep the task within manageable bounds, we have had to omit other important aspects of family health which may be the target of health-promotion activities. Thus we have excluded sex education, information about birth control, promotion of good parenting and family relationships, and building up community links to support parents. Other outcomes that we have not considered include knowledge of health services and appropriate benefits, maternal mental and physical health, satisfaction with maternity care and the experience of childbearing, and the extent to which information needs are met. Clearly, in many interventions and evaluations these outcomes cannot be separated from the 'harder' outcomes that we have concentrated on. Social, psychological and physical wellbeing are interrelated, as are the lives of the family members.[44]

Where we felt that a topic was too large to be dealt with adequately within the confines of this review, we have mentioned it only briefly. In particular, we have taken this approach to the two important topics of sudden infant death and community interventions aimed at supporting new parents. Other topics not covered include pregnancies which are expected to be delivered of multiple births, the special needs of women with physical disabilities, and projects aimed at families who have a child with a particular health problem or disability. Other relevant HEA reviews of health promotion cover childhood accidents and antenatal and postnatal education for first-time parents.[28,45]

1.8 Evaluation criteria

The effects of health-promotion interventions are not always easy to quantify. Observational studies are hard to interpret and trials in this field are difficult to design. Research undertaken to investigate the efficacy of particular interventions has not always been conclusive, even when there are test and control groups. Some trials have failed to assess crucial outcomes, and many trials are methodologically inadequate to some degree. Few health-promotion campaigns occur in isolation, making it difficult to demonstrate substantial differences between intervention and control groups.

This review looks to see whether there are randomised controlled trials which provide reasonably strong evidence about the effects of health-promotion interventions on relevant aspects of behaviour, and on maternal and infant health outcomes. Other types of research are used to provide background information about poor health outcomes and their associations with sociodemographic characteristics and particular behaviours and, more generally, where trials are inappropriate or have not been conducted.

Finally, although sample size has been taken into consideration, no rigid restrictions have been used. Some 'small-scale' studies may be of major importance to health-care providers who try to ensure that they have tailored care provision to the needs of all sections of the community. Small sample sizes are not a problem if the effect of the intervention was so great that a large sample was unnecessary. On the other hand, sample sizes can be restricted if the affected population is small. This can arise when very specific interventions are tailored for use regionally or locally. On other occasions sample sizes are small because of a fault in the study design or because of insufficient funding. Where sample sizes are inappropriate, both positive and negative findings must be interpreted with caution.

Section

2

Lifestyle factors in pregnancy

The health of the developing fetus is affected by the environment in the womb. Many drugs, including nicotine and alcohol, can cross the placenta and may have serious effects on the baby. Some of these may be chronic and debilitating.[46] This section looks at health-promotion activities during pregnancy that aim to promote and support health-enhancing behaviour in women. It covers smoking, illegal drugs, alcohol, diet, work, exercise, and infections in pregnancy. Section 3 deals with health promotion concerned with service use in pregnancy.

The aim of health promotion directed to lifestyle factors in pregnancy is to encourage women to adopt healthy or healthier forms of behaviour. These changes could potentially improve the woman's own health, optimise the fetus's environment and increase the chances of positive pregnancy outcomes. Evidence is needed, though, about the most effective ways of changing behaviour, and about the impact of such interventions on the health of mother and child.

Changing lifestyles requires a great deal of commitment from those who are being asked to make the change. It is therefore necessary that advice is not only based on sound evidence, but is imparted in ways that give women the incentive to make the required effort. Women may be more eager to adapt their lifestyle during pregnancy if they believe that such changes will benefit them and their babies.

2.1 Smoking

Potential impact of health promotion at population level	**High**
Potential impact of health promotion on individuals	**High**
Relevant research	**Yes**
Evidence of impact on behaviour	**Yes**
Evidence of impact on outcomes	**Limited**

Cigarettes introduce significant amounts of chemical substances in the smoker's body. Tobacco smoke includes up to 4000 different types of toxic compounds, including carcinogens heavy metals, and respiratory irritants.[47] Many of these can cross the placenta, influencing the process of fetal development, and may have serious long- and short-term effects on the baby.

Smoking is strongly correlated with poor outcomes in pregnancy. There is evidence that cigarette smoking has harmful effects on the developing fetus, but it is difficult to quantify this as women who are at higher risk for other reasons are also more likely to smoke. Thus, although a statistical dose–response relationship has been derived between smoking and preterm delivery, low birthweight and morbidity in babies,[48] the interpretation of the relationship is not clear-cut. This makes it important to take into account both the direct adverse effects of smoking and the factors confounded with them.

Direct effects

Smoking during pregnancy interferes with the efficiency of the placenta as the blood vessels in the placenta constrict.[48] Smoking during pregnancy is associated with intrauterine growth retardation and shortened gestation, and hence with perinatal mortality and morbidity.[47] Children born to women who smoke are believed to have an increased risk of sudden infant death, asthma, bronchitis and pneumonia,[49] and there is concern that childhood cancers,[47] minimal brain dysfunction and altered central nervous system (CNS) development may also be associated with maternal smoking.[50,51]

Table 2 Prevalence of cigarette smoking in all women by socioeconomic group and economic status (1984–90, Great Britain). *Source:* General Household Survey, 1990.

	Percentage smoking cigarettes				
	1984	1986	1988	1990	(Base)
Socioeconomic group* *(aged 16 or over)*					
I	15	19	17	16	(510)
II	29	27	26	23	(1584)
IIINM	28	27	27	27	(2419)
IIIM	37	36	35	32	(2473)
IV	37	35	37	36	(1690)
V	36	33	39	36	(440)
Economic* status *(aged 16–59 years)†*					
Working full-time	33	34	33	32	(2505)
Working part-time	36	31	33	29	(1967)
All working §	34	32	33	31	(4543)
Unemployed	48	43	44	54	(252)
Inactive	39	38	36	36	(1901)

* = Based on the present job of those in work and last job of those not in work. Married women classified according to their husbands' occupation.

† = Full time students excluded in 1984.

§ = Including a few whose hours of work were unknown.

The prevalence of smoking varies widely within the population and patterns are changing. Although before the 1980s men tended to smoke more than women, women are now just as likely to smoke and are more likely to become persistent smokers.[52] Indeed, in 1990 28 per cent of men and 32 per cent of women between the ages of 16 and 19 years old smoked. Smoking is more common in women with husbands in manual occupations (Table 2). More than twice the proportion of women and three times the number of men from lower socioeconomic groups smoke than do better-off women and men.

Table 3 Proportion of women who smoked before pregnancy, during pregnancy, and who gave up during pregnancy, by socioeconomic group as defined by current or last occupation of husband/ partner (1985 and 1990, Great Britain). *Source:* OPCS (1990) *Infant Feeding*, HMSO.

Socio-economic group	Smoked before pregnancy (%)		Smoked during pregnancy (%)		Smokers who stopped smoking during pregnancy (%)		Number	
	1985	1990	1985	1990	1985	1990	1985	1990
I	16	17	8	8	51	50	307	398
II	26	23	18	13	32	41	1028	1052
IIINM	28	26	19	16	35	41	436	427
IIIM	41	40	31	29	25	37	1666	1611
IV	41	45	32	34	23	24	738	736
V	53	47	46	39	13	17	247	117
Single*	64	62	53	53	17	16	595	760
Uncl†	45	39	38	29	15	26	207	313
Total	39	38	30	28	24	27	5224	5413

* = No partner
† = Unclassified

Data on smoking from the OPCS Infant Feeding surveys show that in 1990, 45 per cent of all women with partners in either partly skilled or unskilled manual occupations smoked cigarettes before their pregnancies, compared with only 17 per cent in professional households[53] (Table 3). During pregnancy, women with partners in professional occupations had the lowest smoking rate (8 per cent), whereas women without partners had the highest rates (53 per cent) (1990, Table 3).[53] White women, those who had lost a partner through bereavement or estrangement, unemployed women and women who lived in deprived areas were also more likely to smoke than other women.[53]

The associations between socioeconomic group and smoking behaviour among women need to be understood if interventions are to be successful at reducing smoking overall. Women who smoke are often the most deprived, even within the family.[54] Among low-income households, women who smoke are more likely to be dependent on income support, are more likely to be lone parents and have greater responsibility than men for managing the home.[55] For many of these women, smoking ceases to be a luxury: it becomes a necessity which provides a way for them to deal with their responsibilities. It is for them 'a way of coping with the constant and unremitting demands of caring: a way of temporarily escaping without leaving the room'.[54] In *The Health of the Nation* the government outlined its targets for combating the harmful effects of smoking generally and during pregnancy as follows:[2]

> '*To reduce the prevalence of cigarette smoking in men and women aged 16 and over to no more than 20 per cent by the year 2000 (a reduction of at least 35 per cent in men and 29 per cent in women, from a prevalence in 1990 of 31 per cent and 28 per cent respectively).*'

and

> '*In addition to the overall reduction in prevalence, at least a third of women smokers to stop smoking at the start of their pregnancy by the year 2000.*'

The government also hopes to reduce the use of cigarettes by 40 per cent at least by the year 2000, from 98 billion cigarettes manufactured in 1990 to 59 billion.

Research on smoking cessation in pregnancy

There has been a large number of studies of interventions to help women give up smoking during pregnancy. Three recent reviews of the relevant randomised controlled trials have been identified. One, by Walsh and Redman, is published in a journal.[56] The second, by Lumley, is contained in an electronic database of controlled trials which is regularly updated.[57] The third is an HEA review on smoking in pregnancy.[58] Two of the reviews use similar methods, with some differences of emphasis, and the third takes a different approach, but all three come to broadly similar conclusions and are used here to report on the stage that research has reached so far.

Anti-smoking interventions covered by the reviews fall into three main types, behavioural strategies, advice and counselling, and feedback.

Behavioural strategies used for reducing smoking have included providing women with a number of assignments or goals which they strive to achieve each week. These encourage women to consider what it is that causes them to smoke, and motivate them towards finding other ways of dealing with those causes. Trials of good methodological quality have been carried out on behavioural strategies and have shown that they are more effective than advice or counselling.

Trials on advice and counselling for giving up smoking are of 'mixed' methodological quality.[57] Advice for the intervention groups was largely given on a one-to-one basis during pregnancy, or with a pamphlet supplemented by advice from the person giving antenatal care. Although advice did reduce the number of women who continued to smoke throughout pregnancy, the effect was small. In the only trial which focused exclusively on the efficacy of counselling,[59] only 10 per cent of the participants received all or part of the intervention. No assessment could therefore be made on the benefits of counselling on either an individualised or a group basis. Overall, brief advice from general practitioners during routine consultations is more effective than no advice in helping a small but significant number of smokers to stop for at least a year.

Reviewers differed in their assessment of trials using feedback methods for stopping smoking. Three trials and three different forms of feedback were identified. These were: telling women about their carbon monoxide level;[60,61] telling them about the effects of smoking on birthweight;[61] and feedback about the fetus during an early ultrasound examination.[62] The results showed that feedback about the fetus was associated with a significant reduction in the proportion of women who continued to smoke during the next six weeks of the pregnancy. Longer-term results were not assessed. On the other hand, feedback about carbon monoxide levels and about the probable effects of cotinine results on birthweight are both difficult to assess because of methodological problems with the relevant trials.

Putting effective interventions into practice

Two of the reviews[56,58] emphasise the need to find interventions that are not only effective but also practical to apply in normal care situations. They draw attention to the fact that many of the trials use extra personnel, such as health educators, and that these staff would not normally be available. The HEA review recommends that the most promising behavioural interventions be tested in the UK in methodologically sound controlled trials that are based on normal health-service provision.

Summary

Taking together all the aspects of smoking cessation, we can draw some broad conclusions. On the present evidence, behavioural self-help strategies seem to be most effective in helping women to stop smoking during pregnancy, but how effective are they at producing longer-term abstinence? In terms of the main outcomes of importance for this review, the research shows that interventions aimed at reducing smoking lead to a small increase in average birthweight, but so far have not been shown to reduce perinatal mortality, preterm delivery or the proportion of babies of low birthweight.[57]

There is the possibility that anti-smoking interventions may have some adverse consequences for those who do not stop. Pregnant women who fail to give up may continue to smoke, with the added burdens of guilt and anxiety[63,64] and feelings of inadequacy.[65] Trials could look at these outcomes and at ways of maximising the benefits of smoking cessation programmes.

2.2 Illegal drugs

Potential impact of health promotion at population level	**Low in UK**
Potential impact of health promotion on individuals	**High**
Relevant research	**Little**
Evidence of impact on behaviour	**Virtually none**
Evidence of impact on outcomes	**No**

The use of illegal drugs such as cocaine by women of childbearing age increased markedly in the USA in the late 1970s and early 1980s.[66] They are not widely used in the UK, but these substances are known to have many very harmful effects on both mother and child. It is possible that the use of habit-forming drug taking is on the increase among young women. Although the effects of alcohol and nicotine on pregnancy outcome are widely reported, fewer data are available on street drugs such as marijuana and heroin.[67] In addition to the increased risk of contracting HIV if drugs are injected with shared equipment, illegal drug use during pregnancy is believed to be implicated in preterm birth[68,69] and still birth,[70] has an effect on fetal growth and birthweight,[71] and may predispose exposed babies to a higher risk of sudden infant deaths.[72] The best evidence of the efficacy of interventions will come from work on non-pregnant groups. If these are found to be effective, they could be adapted for use with pregnant women.

2.3 Alcohol

Potential impact of health promotion at population level	**Probably low in UK**
Potential impact of health promotion on individuals	**High**
Relevant research	**Some**
Evidence of impact on behaviour	**Yes**
Evidence of impact on outcomes	**No**

Both intoxication and regular excessive alcohol use can cause physical and social damage[73,74] and is costly in terms of death and illness and sickness absence.[75] In addition to these general dangers, the use of alcohol during pregnancy appears to have adverse effects on fetal growth: consumption of two or more drinks a day is related to a decrease in birthweight.[76-80] Excessive alcohol consumption in pregnancy can lead to fetal alcohol syndrome (FAS), a combination of conditions which includes growth retardation, mental retardation and facial dysmorphology. Affected babies may also exhibit altered neonatal behaviour. The severity of signs and symptoms may vary between babies.[76,79] The incidence of FAS in Britain is not known; some researchers suggest that it is between one and four per 1000 live births,[81] while others describe FAS as 'rare'.[77,82] In North America, figures are believed to be between 1.3 and 2.2 per 1000 live births.[83] The use of alcohol by pregnant women who also smoke appears to compound the effects of smoking, possibly by inhibiting the deposition of fat in the fetus and thereby contributing to the reduction in birthweight associated with these activities.[66]

There is a debate about whether pregnant women should be advised to avoid alcohol completely,[78,84] which has arisen because different epidemiological studies have reached different conclusions about the effects of low to moderate drinking in pregnancy. This is a problem common to many such attempts to link behaviour and outcomes, and arises partly because lifestyle factors and other characteristics of women are associated, so that it is hard to make causal links. At present, pregnant women in the UK are advised to avoid alcohol if possible, or to aim at consumption of no more than one or two units a week.[31] A recent European Concerted Action on alcohol in pregnancy[78] recommended that women avoid alcohol if possible, or alternatively limit themselves to no more than one standard drink a day. There is evidence from animal studies to support advice to women to avoid sudden high intakes of alcohol (binge drinking).[78]

Drinking trends

General Household Survey data from 1984 onwards show that a higher proportion of women than men in Britain are non-drinkers, and that women who do drink consume less than men.[52] This holds true over all age groups. In the 1990 OPCS Infant Feeding Survey, 86 per cent of all mothers used alcohol before their pregnancies, while 67 per cent continued to drink while pregnant.[53] Of these women, 99 per cent drank less than the recommended weekly maximum for women who are not pregnant (15 units) with 72 per cent drinking less than one unit per week.

Table 4 shows clear class differences in drinking habits but, unlike smoking, women from socioeconomic group I were more likely than those from groups IV and V to drink alcohol before pregnancy. Women from non-manual classes were also more likely than the others to drink less than one unit per week.[53] The sample was not large enough to produce separate figures for minority ethnic groups.

Table 4 Estimated weekly alcohol consumption of mothers who drank during pregnancy, by socioeconomic group as defined by current or last occupation of husband/partner (1990, Great Britain). *Source:* OPCS (1990) *Infant Feeding*, HMSO

Socioeconomic group	Percentage who drank during pregnancy				No. of women in sample
	Less than 1 unit	1–7 units	8–14 units	15 or more units	
I	73	25	2	0	278
II	76	22	2	1	752
IIINM	76	23	1	0	295
IIIM	71	25	3	1	1095
IV	71	25	3	2	463
V	68	28	3	2	74
Np*	64	27	6	2	506
Uncl†	78	17	4	1	179
Total	72	24	3	1	3642

* = No Partner

† = Unclassified

Research on drinking in pregnancy

Research has attempted to evaluate health strategies to reduce alcohol use during pregnancy.[84,85] Two trials conducted in England looked at three methods of giving information in the antenatal clinic, designed to reduce alcohol consumption during pregnancy.[86] Women participating in these trials were not selected because they had a problem with alcohol use. In the first trial, 477 women were provided with written information at their booking clinic and compared with another 559 who were given the written information plus advice from the doctor. In the second trial, written information (the same as that used in the first trial) was provided for 564 women, while another 500 received the written information and the same medical advice as well as watching a specially produced video on alcohol use in pregnancy. The researchers found no evidence that any of the interventions was effective in changing drinking behaviour. Women in both groups from the second trial were more likely than those in the first trial to say that they should not use more than one unit of alcohol daily. The authors suggest that external factors, such as information given in the mass media, may have increased awareness while failing to induce behavioural changes. They conclude that special and expensive arrangements for alcohol reduction in pregnancy are not necessary in the antenatal clinic, but that appropriate advice could be incorporated into existing antenatal educational programmes.

Health-promotion advice about the use of alcohol during pregnancy, as found in *The Pregnancy Book* is probably appropriate based on current knowledge.

Nevertheless, effective interventions are needed to help the smaller numbers of women who are heavy drinkers. Interventions that are found to be effective for the non-pregnant population should be adapted and tested for pregnant women. A recent review[87] of research on general populations concluded first, that simple screening tests used in routine clinical settings can pick up people drinking above the recommended level, and second, that brief (and cheap) interventions can be effective in reducing drinking by over 20 per cent.

Waterson and Murray-Lyon[84] suggest that women should be asked about their drinking habits at their first antenatal clinic, so that excessive drinkers can be identified and appropriate advice given. Screening is quick and cheap, but evidence from the Infant Feeding Survey,[53] and from trials,[84,85] suggests that only a very small percentage of pregnant women drink more than the recommended amount. It would be useful to investigate further the costs and benefits of introducing this process into routine antenatal care in different settings in the UK.

2.4 Diet

Impact of health promotion at population level	**Moderate on present evidence**
Potential impact of health promotion on individuals	**Varies depending on aspect of diet**
Relevant research	**Extensive but patchy**
Evidence of impact on behaviour	**Yes**
Evidence of impact on outcomes	**Likely to be limited**

There is growing interest in the relationship between maternal nutrition and human fetal growth and development. Evidence from epidemiological studies shows a relationship between maternal diet and pregnancy outcome in times of severe food restriction: in Third World countries[88] and in Europe during famine conditions, severely malnourished women were found to have babies of reduced birthweight.[89-92] However, as already indicated, birthweight is affected by a range of factors, including maternal age, parity, smoking habits, illness and placental adequacy, which may obscure the relationship between maternal diet and birthweight in populations where frank malnutrition is rare.

Although there is evidence to suggest that poor outcomes are associated with low prepregnancy weight and poor weight gain in pregnancy,[93] investigators in developed countries have found only weak correlations or no significant correlations between maternal diet and weight gain and between maternal diet and birthweight. Among the most vulnerable groups of women improvements in diet may result in improvements in birthweight;[94] however, on the basis of evidence from randomised trials, the enhancements in fetal growth to be expected from energy and protein supplementation for pregnant women are modest and without important long-term benefits for child growth and development.[95]

None the less, inadequacies or excessive intake of certain nutrients during pregnancy have also been associated with a range of other perinatal problems. These include biochemical deficiencies,[96] intellectual and behavioural development[97] and teratogenesis. In addition, the work of Barker[98,99] suggests that there may be links with increased risk of cardiovascular disease in later life. Health-promotion advice about diet in pregnancy needs to reflect these concerns.

Current recommendations in the UK for diet during pregnancy are now briefly reviewed with respect to the risk of adverse outcomes, evidence of benefits associated with intervention and identification of vulnerable groups.

Dietary recommendations

Energy

Evidence from surveys in the Five-Country Study[100] and Holland[101] indicate that the additional energy requirements of pregnancy, associated with satisfactory outcomes, among such populations are probably modest. Consequently, it is recommended[102] that an additional 0.8 MJ/day (200 kcal/day) above the estimated average requirement (EAR) during the last trimester should meet the needs of most women, although those who are underweight at the beginning of pregnancy or do not reduce their activity levels as pregnancy progresses may need more.

Protein

The most recent recommendations for the UK[102] proposed an additional 6g/day above the reference nutrient intake (RNI) throughout pregnancy.

Meta-analysis of published trials[95] indicates that trials of balanced energy and protein supplementation have demonstrated only modest increases in maternal weight gain and fetal growth, even in undernourished women, and no long-term benefits to the child in terms of growth or neurocognitive development. Neither balanced isoenergetic protein supplementation nor high-protein supplementation appears beneficial to either mother or infant, and may even impair fetal growth.

Vitamins

At the present time, evidence suggests that, as a result of the normal physiological processes of adaptation to pregnancy, requirements for thiamin, niacin and vitamin B_6 are not increased during pregnancy. For the majority of omnivorous women there is no need to increase intake of vitamin B_{12} during pregnancy either. However, those whose body stores are depleted at the outset of pregnancy, or who are following a strict vegetarian/vegan diet, may be at increased risk of megaloblastic anaemia. At present there are no dietary reference values for pantothenic acid, biotin, vitamin E or vitamin K, owing to a lack of data.

Vitamin A

During pregnancy extra vitamin A is required for the growth and maintenance of the fetus, to provide it with some reserves and for maternal tissue growth, hence the raised RNI of 700 µg/day. Most women have a normal intake in excess of this and only a small number are likely to require supplementary vitamin A during pregnancy. In fact, in view of the teratogenic potential of vitamin A,[103] it is recommended by the Teratology Society[104] that supplementation should be limited to 8000 IU (2400 µg) a day. This advice has been reiterated in even stronger terms by the Chief Medical Officer[105] – women in the UK who are, or may become, pregnant have been advised not to take supplements containing Vitamin A unless advised to do so by a doctor or antenatal clinic.

Folate

Even in otherwise well-fed western societies the widespread occurrence of bone marrow megaloblastosis before folate supplementation in pregnancy became widespread during the 1960s[106,107] provides evidence for increased folate requirements in late pregnancy, with the result that women were advised to increase folic acid intake to 0.3 mg/day during pregnancy.[102] However, in the light of evidence suggesting that periconceptual folate supplementation may not only reduce the recurrence of neural tube defects (NTD)[108,109] but also reduce the first occurrence of these defects,[110–112] the Department of Health made further recommendations[113] that all women likely to become pregnant should increase their intake of folic acid by eating more folate-rich foods and foods fortified with folic acid. Women who have not previously had a child with NTD, but who are planning a pregnancy, are also advised to take 0.4 mg/day folic acid (which is available without prescription) for the first 12 weeks of their pregnancy. In the USA the Food and Drug Administration is considering the fortification of appropriate foods with folic acid.[114]

Except under a physician's direction, women should keep their consumption of folic acid below 1 mg/day because of the risk of complicating the diagnosis of pernicious anaemia.[115] However, the Department of Health[113] recommends that women who have previously had a child with NTD should be prescribed a daily dose of 5 mg folic acid (or 4 mg when such a tablet is licensed).

Vitamin C

In its most recent recommendations the Department of Health[102] proposes that increasing the RNI by 10 mg/day during the third trimester is sufficient to meet the increased demands of pregnancy. Earlier suggestions that high doses of ascorbic acid might be teratogenic have been discounted by subsequent work in which daily doses of up to 1000 mg/kg body weight had no effect on embryonic, fetal or postpartum development in four animal species.[116]

Vitamin D

Pregnant women should receive supplementary vitamin D to achieve an intake of 10 mg/day, according to current recommendations.[102] This reflects concern about the higher incidence of hypocalcaemia, hyperparathyroidism and a defect of dental enamel related to vitamin D deficiency in the infants of women not taking vitamin D supplements.[117] Intakes of vitamin D among Asian women have attracted particular attention (see below).

Minerals

In the majority of instances maternal adaptation is considered to ensure that the requirements of both fetus and mother are met during pregnancy.[102] Only in the cases of calcium and iron is there some debate about the need for increased intake during pregnancy.

Calcium

The Department of Health accepts the view that mobilisation of maternal calcium depots, rather than an increase in dietary intake, is an appropriate source of the additional calcium needed for fetal growth,[118] together with increased efficiency of calcium absorption. However, higher maternal intakes are advisable in adolescent pregnancy, where two risk factors combine[119] (see below). In addition, a review of studies of routine supplementation with calcium[120] suggested an association with a reduction in hypertension, proteinuric pre-eclampsia and preterm delivery, although at this moment the available evidence of benefits was promising but inconclusive.

Iron

Although women of childbearing age should have sufficient iron stores to meet the increased demands of pregnancy, when iron stores are low at the start of pregnancy supplementation may be necessary.[102] A substantial body of evidence[121] supports the view that routine supplementation with iron is not appropriate in generally well-nourished populations. However, there may be groups within the population, such as Asian and adolescent mothers, who may benefit from supplementation (see below).

Diet for vulnerable groups

Low income mothers

Although the effects may be modest, there is still some evidence to suggest that improvement in the diets of pregnant women from the most deprived population groups of developed countries can bring changes in outcome. A review in the USA of pregnancy outcomes in the Women, Infants and Children (WIC) program for over 11 million births, estimated that the effect of supplemental food was to increase birthweight by 23 g on average and by 46.6 g for 'less educated whites'. There was also a significant reduction of 1.5 per cent in birthweights less than 2500 g among 'less-educated blacks'.[94] It is therefore of concern that there is evidence that some pregnant women in the UK have diets that do not meet recommendations for adult, non-pregnant women.[122,123] In a further study of women on low incomes, Doyle et al.[124] found low birthweight to be significantly associated with poor intakes of thiamin, riboflavin, niacin, zinc and iron during the first trimester of pregnancy. This effect was to a substantial extent, but not wholly, independent of the effect of prepregnancy weight, and the two effects were cumulative. For this reason, Nelson[125] expressed concern that a Department of Health recommendation[105] to avoid liver would discourage women from consuming a food which is a cheap, rich source of these nutrients (as well as folate and vitamin B_{12}), since on a population basis the risk associated with an inadequate diet was likely to be far greater than the risk associated with vitamin A toxicity. A study in Belfast[126] not only identified the poor diets of low-income pregnant women, but also that few of the subjects were given advice about nutrition early in pregnancy.

Both for their own health and for that of their infants, it would seem that women from low-income groups can be considered an appropriate target group for health-promotion activities focused on improved nutrition, both preconception and during pregnancy.

Adolescent mothers

The particular needs of pregnant adolescents are unclear. However, it has been suggested that since pregnancy and adolescence are both times of rapid growth, nutritional requirements are likely to be increased in pregnant adolescents above those of pregnancy in a fully mature woman. In practice the picture may be further complicated by the sometimes erratic eating habits of adolescents and the disadvantageous social circumstances in which a pregnant teenager may find herself. Endres et al.[127] have expressed concern that if the nutritional reserves of the adolescent have been depleted by poor diet, she will be ill-prepared for pregnancy. Several studies in the USA[128,129] have documented that the intake and serum levels of certain nutrients are lower than those of pregnant adults, and commonly documented deficiencies include vitamins A, C and folate and minerals such as calcium, iron and zinc. This appears to reflect the paucity of dairy products and green leafy vegetables in many adolescent diets.

Teenagers are more likely to be underweight at the beginning of pregnancy and to gain less than 16 lb during pregnancy, which appears to contribute to the outcome of pregnancy in the USA where 19 per cent of infants born to teenagers weigh less than 2500 g.[130] Competition for nutrients as a result of maternal growth during pregnancy has been identified as at least a partial explanation of the differences in birthweight in three studies.[130-132] However, a review of the evidence concerning adolescent weight gain and low birthweight[133] has questioned the benefits of increasing maternal weight gain targets for adolescents, but suggested that intervention would be better directed at correcting deficiencies of iron, calcium and folic acid in the diet.

Mothers from ethnic minorities

Asian

Although studies have shown that babies born to Asian women in the UK are lighter on average by 150–350 g than those born to Caucasian women in the same area, it is uncertain whether this is due to genetic factors or to poor maternal nutrition.[134] The trend towards increasing birthweights over a period of ten years would suggest that genetic factors are not the major cause of these differences.[135] Changes in factors such as longer birth intervals and fewer teenage pregnancies may all play a part.

A number of studies have been undertaken to examine the adequacy of the diets of pregnant Asian women which suggest that the intakes of some nutrients may be lower than those of Caucasian women, although no adverse consequences for the mother or fetus have been demonstrated.[136-138]. However, it is important to distinguish between different groups from the Indian subcontinent. Although energy intakes below recommended levels have been reported for all groups, some studies have shown differences between Sikhs, Hindus, Pakistanis and Bangladeshis. A study carried out in Birmingham[138] reported that Sikhs had the highest intakes of energy and most nutrients, while Bangladeshi women had the lowest except for protein. All groups in this study had below the recommended intake of zinc, copper, vitamin B_{12}, riboflavin and vitamin D, although there was no obvious relationship between dietary intake and fetal growth.

Concern about the risks of neonatal hypocalcaemia and rickets resulting from vitamin D deficiency during pregnancy prompted the Stop Rickets Campaign discussed in Section 3. However, there is probably a continuing need to emphasise the importance of vitamin D intake, as well as vitamin B_{12} and folate, in health promotion designed for Asian groups. More recently, concern has been expressed about the effect of fasting by some pregnant Moslem women during Ramadan,[139] but no effects of this practice on pregnancy outcomes have been demonstrated.

Other minority ethnic groups

Pregnant women with sickle-cell conditions are often deficient in folic acid.[140] In view of the importance of periconceptual folate status identified previously, health-promotion activities in the African–Caribbean community should particularly emphasise the importance of supplementation with folate. The value of routine iron supplementation in well-nourished populations has already been questioned, but in some groups iron supplementation is considered undesirable. Women with sickle-cell conditions and from other ethnic minority groups with thalassaemia, may receive regular blood transfusions during their pregnancies and iron supplementation is not recommended to avoid the possible problem of iron overload.

Effectiveness of health-promotion strategies designed to change eating habits in pregnancy

Having considered nutritional factors which may affect the outcome of pregnancy, it is necessary to consider the available evidence concerning the effectiveness of health-promotion strategies designed to encourage dietary practices that reflect this nutritional advice. Do women change their eating behaviour? Is this reflected in pregnancy outcome? As with so many areas of health promotion the number of well-conducted evaluation studies is limited. In addition, the common observation that it is possible to change knowledge without changing behaviour is reported.[141-143] The authors of a study in Aberdeen[144] emphasise the need to focus on attitudes and beliefs rather than concentrating on information transfer alone.

Nutritional advice given on a one-to-one basis or in groups

A review of the literature[95] found evidence from four prospective controlled studies that nutritional advice given in groups or on a one-to one basis resulted in increased protein and energy intakes. Only one of these studies looked at weight gain in pregnancy and outcome.[145] Maternal weight gain was significantly greater in the intervention group, with some indications of increases in birthweight and reductions in pre-term births. However, the influence of maternal diet on outcomes of pregnancy that occur with low frequency (i.e. low birthweight, neonatal morbidity and neonatal deaths) was hard to interpret in these subjects, who were not nutritionally at risk. In a retrospective study[146] the effectiveness of a one-off group antenatal session was compared with outcomes when mothers had not only attended a group session but also received personalised counselling at every visit. No evidence is presented concerning changes in eating habits, but weight gain was significantly higher in the group who were intensively counselled and there were fewer low-birthweight babies in that group. Subjects in this study were drawn from relatively deprived groups and conclusions are limited by the design, However, the findings accord with expectations from other research that the most vulnerable groups are more likely to show a change in pregnancy outcome, and that personalised health advice is more effective. Properly controlled prospective interventions need to be undertaken to establish whether this would be useful approach to intervention in the UK.

Listeriosis and other foodborne infections

Good food hygiene practices are always important, but recent publicity has focused particular attention on the hazards of listeria and salmonella in foods and the risks to pregnant women. Infection with these organisms can result in miscarriage, still birth and maternal death. Listeria is found in many foods; those that present a particular hazard include raw chicken, precooked ready-to-eat poultry and other chilled meats and soft cheeses such as Brie and blue-veined cheeses.[147] In 1989 The Department of Health advised pregnant women to avoid certain soft cheeses, all types of paté and to heat all cook–chill foods until they are 'piping hot'[148] in order to reduce the risk of listeriosis. However, the evidence on which this advice was based is very limited and the small numbers of women likely to be affected make attempts to evaluate health-promotion activities very difficult.

Foodborne infection with salmonella has received considerable publicity, focused on the risk of contaminated eggs and products in which raw egg is an ingredient, such as mayonnaise. However, other foods, particularly poultry and meat when improperly cooked, are also common sources of infection. This serves to emphasise that health-promotion advice in pregnancy should reinforce the general messages about personal and food hygiene and thorough cooking which are important for the whole UK population in the light of the increasing levels of illness due to foodborne pathogens.

Advice on diet and pre-eclampsia

Pre-eclampsia can occur from about 20 weeks' gestation onwards and may affect as many as one in ten of all pregnancies.[149] It is characterised by hypertension, proteinuria and oedema, and poses serious risks to both mother and baby.[150]

Studies in the past have suggested that body weight and diet are important determinants of whether a woman is likely to develop pre-eclampsia during pregnancy.[151,152] There have also been suggestions that the use of small amounts of aspirin during pregnancy could prevent pre-eclampsia,[153] and a large-scale trial, the CLASP trial, is currently under way. In addition, women with early signs of impending pre-eclampsia are advised to rest in bed and encouraged to relax as much as possible.

One difficulty in interpreting trials and other work on pre-eclampsia is that researchers have varied in the ways in which they have defined pre-eclampsia, pregnancy-induced hypertension and toxaemia. This has made it difficult to make comparisons. In any case, the trials were generally of medical interventions to deal with these conditions rather than health promotion to prevent them.

There have been no trials since the mid 1980s, so advice on diet in pregnancy is based on earlier research. The best-known study of the effects of diet on pre-eclampsia is of the Dutch famine during World War II.[154] This study showed a fall in the incidence of hypertension, pre-eclampsia and eclampsia when the calorific intake of pregnant women who were previously well-nourished fell to around 600 calories per day, compared with the periods before and after the famine. Even the poorest women in Britain do not live under such conditions and are comparatively well nourished. Studies done more recently, but published before 1985, have tended to involve well-nourished women and have been poorly controlled for some of the other variables which could have an effect on pre-eclampsia, such as age and parity.[155]

Obesity is now seen as a proven risk factor for the development of pre-eclampsia,[151] despite the lack of clear proof that diet as a whole, or even average or low intakes of one or more of its constituent components, such as protein, salt, calories and vitamins, can affect a pregnant woman's chance of developing pre-eclampsia.[150]

2.5 Employment and pregnancy

Potential impact of health promotion
  at population level................................. **Probably low**
Potential impact of health promotion
  on individuals .... **Possibly high**
Relevant research .... **Very little**
Evidence of impact on behaviour .... **No**
Evidence of impact on outcomes................ **No**

There is no evidence from epidemiological studies that participation in paid work is, *per se*, a problem for pregnant women. In fact, it may offer some advantages because of increased confidence and social contact. Studies of this kind are difficult to interpret, however, because women in employment differ in many ways from those without paid work, and studies in different countries come up with different associations.[156-160]

Some types of workplace, industry or work itself (such as the use of a production line, physical effort, night work or long hours) are thought to be linked with poor pregnancy outcomes. Research is very difficult to conduct and interpret because women with other disadvantages may also find themselves doing hard or unpleasant work, and because the industries that have caused concern[161,162] generally employ very few women.

Health promotion is very limited in relation to the safe employment of pregnant women, although some trades unions and occupational health workers may give specific advice to those for whom they are responsible. Women are likely to find it hard to obtain good advice because of the limited knowledge so far. Reliable studies that evaluate either changes in work organisation for pregnant women or health-promotion interventions in this field have not been found.

2.6 Recreational exercise

Potential impact of health promotion at population level	**Low**
Potential impact of health promotion on individuals	**Possibly high**
Relevant research	**Some small trials of exercise, other observational studies; limited value**
Evidence of impact on behaviour	**No clear basis for HP advice**
Evidence of impact on outcomes	**No clear basis for HP advice**

Although only a small proportion of pregnant women are likely to be taking regular vigorous recreational exercise, the issue of fitness is relevant to all. Pregnancy may provide an opportunity to encourage women to become more active and this is likely to be of benefit to them. Although the effect on pregnancy outcome of moderate intensity activity is not known, data available indicate that it is beneficial for most women if appropriate guidelines are followed. The most commonly asked and researched question is whether vigorous activity is harmful to the developing fetus and likely to lead to a poor outcome. Although there is a considerable number of small-scale studies, only a few have been methodologically satisfactory. One review of 18 studies of physical exercise in pregnancy[163] concluded that vigorous exercise did not have an adverse effect on the measures of pregnancy outcome included in the studies, but unfortunately included non-randomised comparisons in its meta-analysis. A recent review of the relevant randomised controlled trials[164] found that there was not enough evidence to draw conclusions about the effects of exercise on pregnancy outcomes. Larger trials which looked at a range of outcomes were recommended to give far clearer guidance about the positive and negative effects of recreational exercise.

2.7 Infections in pregnancy

Potential impact of health promotion at population level	**Probably limited in UK**
Potential impact of health promotion on individuals	**Great**
Relevant research	**Limited**
Evidence of impact on behaviour	**One relevant study**
Evidence of impact on outcomes	**Not so far**

Infection during pregnancy may lead to maternal and infant mortality and morbidity.[165-168] There has been more concern about infection in pregnancy in North America than in the UK, and there has been extensive research on the possible effects of sexually transmitted and other infections. The possible role of infection in preterm delivery means that this may prove to be an important area in the future for both medical and health-promotion intervention. In the UK, maternal infection is probably not a major cause of poor pregnancy outcomes, but this conclusion may need to be revised.

Preventive measures are used to avoid the problems of rubella infection and are largely successful in the general population. Between 1974 and 1984, congenital rubella was 2–3 times higher in Asian births than in other births in England and Wales[8]. This was believed to be because many of the women involved were first-generation immigrants arriving too late to receive routine school immunisation, and their first contact with the health services followed conception.[169,170] Since then, a programme of immunisation has been carried out and this has been promoted through health-promotion campaigns for Asian women. No research assessing the effectiveness of rubella immunisation programmes for Asian women has been found.

Other types of infection may be amenable to health-promotion interventions but continue to be problematic, as many women may not even be aware that they have been infected.[171,172] Many of these infections may only be noticed up during routine screening, when it becomes apparent that all is not well with the fetus[171] or if a woman is suspected of having a potentially serious infection.[172] Much of the research on infection in pregnancy focused on medical rather than health promotion interventions. Only one study of a health-promotion intervention for toxoplasmosis has been identified.

Toxoplasmosis may affect pregnant women at the rate of between two and six per 1000,[172, 173] and may affect anything from 40 to 560 babies per annum.[172, 174] No studies on health promotion in the UK were identified, but an education programme developed in Canada specifically to reduce the risk of congenital toxoplasmosis, has been evaluated in a randomised controlled trial.[175] The programme was successful in changing self-reported behaviour, and the study indicates that education programmes that highlight the risks to the fetus of pet, personal and food hygiene are acceptable to pregnant women and can have a positive effect on hygiene behaviours. However, it is not clear whether these results were also associated with a decrease in the incidence of toxoplasmosis.

Section 3

Service use in pregnancy

This section covers attempts to influence the uptake of professional care, in order to reduce perceived risks to the pregnancy. For example, books and leaflets advise women to seek care in pregnancy and discuss the likely pattern of care. We look at routine care and then at projects directed to special groups within the population. There follows a section on genetic screening. Although relatively little experimental work has been done on either the effectiveness of systems of antenatal care, or on the success of the specific aspects of health promotion in pregnancy, some relevant evaluations are available and are described below.

3.1 Antenatal care

Potential impact of health promotion at population level	**Limited in the UK**
Potential impact of health promotion on individuals	**High**
Relevant research	**Little research on health-promotion interventions about antenatal attendance in the UK**
Evidence of impact on behaviour	**No**
Evidence of impact on outcomes	**No**

Although there have been systematic evaluations of many of the clinical components of antenatal care there has been less attention directed to the whole pattern of care.[176-179] In countries where maternity care is either inaccessible or too expensive, there are important potential benefits of attendance to women and their babies.[176] In western Europe, although the timing and number of visits vary considerably between and within countries, there are generally relatively few women who receive little or no care.[177] In the UK there has been a general recognition that efforts should be directed to further assessment of the effectiveness of the clinical components of care, to reducing needless duplication and rationalising the schedule of visits, and to making care more convenient, acceptable and supportive to women.[178-180]

There are concerns here about getting the appropriate parts of the antenatal 'package' to those who need them, for example by ensuring that women make contact with the services in time to benefit from tests. This is a complex area, because the technology and use of the relevant tests (such as ultrasound or chorion villus sampling) is evolving, and because research about the benefits and hazards of the tests is incomplete.[181,182] Some categories of women may particularly benefit from early attendance (see below). Some research about women who attend late for antenatal care is discussed in the HEA review of antenatal and postnatal education.[28] Women from minority groups, including African–Caribbeans, have been reported as booking late for care during their pregnancies.[183-187] Where booking takes place in hospital, some studies of late booking have indicated that part of the delay is due to late referral by GPs.[184-189]

Apart from steps to improve the accessibility and quality of care and to encourage GPs to refer women promptly, there are unlikely to be significant health gains in non-specific health promotion aimed at bringing women in earlier for care. This may not be true for interventions targeted at particular subgroups of women, however. In addition, the opportunity for general health promotion presented by antenatal care should not be ignored.

3.2 Care for special groups

There is clear evidence of inequalities in the health of mothers. Some women, including very young mothers and mothers from minority ethnic groups (including traveller mothers), have particularly poor health despite the apparent availability of extensive maternity services.[190-193] Furthermore, there are wide variations in the efforts made to meet the needs of subgroups of the population.[186,194,195]

Minority ethnic communities

Potential impact of health promotion
  at population level .... **Uncertain, service provision needs to change before major health promotion**

Potential impact of health promotion
  on individuals .... **High**

Relevant research .... **A little**

Evidence of impact on behaviour .... **Asian Mother and Baby Campaign**

Evidence of impact on outcomes .... **No**

The Stop Rickets Campaign launched in 1979 highlighted the problems many Asian women had in making use of the health services.[196] This led to a Department of Health/Save the Children Fund initiative to improve the health of Asian mothers and babies. The Asian Mother and Baby Campaign (AMBC), launched in 1984, had two main thrusts. First, there was a programme of publicity and health promotion. Second, link workers who were fluent in English and at least one Asian language were employed to facilitate the interactions between health workers and their clients. The AMBC's aims were to encourage early diagnosis of pregnancy and uptake of maternity services; to improve communication between mothers and health professionals; to help health professionals gain the cooperation of Asian families; to help Asian families to become more aware of the services, and to ensure that the services provided were accessible and acceptable.

An evaluation of the AMBC by the University of Leicester discussed a number of interesting points and findings.[197-200] Although using local media and activities to promote the campaign was deemed appropriate, it was found that the publicity had very limited success in making Asian women aware of the scheme. This might have been because the material was somewhat general and did not target those likely to be actively interested in the campaign.[199]

In general the link-worker scheme seemed to be successful, with improvements being made to several aspects of client care. These included the provision of more antenatal, parentcraft and family planning classes for Asian women, improved quality of information generally, and improvements in the quality and continuity of care.[199] Although link workers were seen as providing a much-needed interpreter service, they were less successful at imparting health education knowledge to Asian women.[200]

The evaluation suggested that the campaign was also weakened by a lack of specific objectives, which initially allowed structural racism to be ignored. Protests by the community and growing evidence of racism led the campaign to place greater emphasis on these problems, which would largely be faced by and have an effect on the role of link workers. There were difficulties regarding their management. For example, it was not clear to whom link workers should be accountable. It was also unclear whether they were to be interpreters or advocates. Link workers were seen to be more confident at tackling racist attitudes after they had undergone a period of training on race awareness.

The AMBC raises the issue of the type of health promotion that should be aimed at groups within the population for whom adequate services do not exist. Few women who do not speak English have access to link workers or interpreters in the course of their maternity care.[201] There is also evidence that some Asian women have unmet needs for information about childbearing and maternity care.[201]

Another project which examined meeting the needs of minority ethnic groups was the experiment in advocacy which was carried out in Hackney.[187] This project had similar aims to the AMBC and focused on the needs of Asian and Turkish women. Here the advocates had very clearly defined roles, including giving 'health education and antenatal talks, taking information when women first booked in, staying with women who had difficult labours and a range of other activities'.[195]

The project was seen to be successful in a number of ways,[187,195] including significant changes in the 'antenatal length of stay, induction and mode of delivery'. There were seen to be reductions in antenatal stay from 8.6 to 5.7 days and a fall in caesarean rates from 10.8 per cent to 8.5 per cent. Although these changes cannot be directly attributed to health advocacy, improved communication could have improved clinical practice. Thus, health advocacy may offer a mechanism to address some of the adverse obstetric outcomes observed in minority ethnic groups.

3.3 Genetic screening

Potential impact of health promotion
   on population level................................. **Fairly low**
Potential impact of health promotion
   on individuals....................................... **High**
Relevant research.................................... **Background, yes; health
                                                       promotion, no**
Evidence of impact on behaviour................. **No**
Evidence of impact on outcomes .... **No**

Antenatal screening for fetal abnormalities and other identifiable genetic conditions that lead to mortality and morbidity among babies is a feature of most antenatal care in the industrialised world.[202] Tests that may be offered during pregnancy include ultrasound scanning, amniocentesis, chorionic villus sampling and alphafetoprotein (AFP). Although congenital anomalies play a significant part in still birth and infant mortality, not all conditions are amenable to prenatal diagnosis.

Compared with younger women, women nearing the end of their childbearing years have a greater risk of having babies with chromosomal abnormalities, such as Down's syndrome.[203] Others possess particular genotypes which may lead to an increased risk of mortality or chronic illness and disability in their babies. It is known that some ethnic groups are more at risk than others of particular kinds of genetic disease, such as the haemoglobinopathies, Tay–Sachs disease, Duchenne muscular dystrophy and haemophilia.[204-206] Furthermore, some ethnic groups who practise customary consanguineous marriage may have higher perinatal mortality due to an increased incidence of congenital malformations.[207,208] However, the results of early studies are unreliable because of a failure to control for other factors affecting congenital abnormality.[209] There are complex and interrelated factors affecting these groups, who may also be at increased risk for other reasons.[209]

Although all pregnant women attending antenatal clinics in Britain undergo some form of screening, age, race and known carrier status for particular genes are identifiable risk factors. The specific goals of antenatal screening are first, to identify fetuses which are at risk, secondly to inform women and their partners of that risk, and thirdly to offer them counselling, which would include choices they could make that could have an effect on the future outcome of the pregnancy.[205,210,211]

Research has shown that people who are carriers of recessive genes which have no adverse effects on the carrier's health have less optimistic views of their future health.[212,213] Prospective parents may not be informed of the risk to their babies or given any professional support in exploring strategies which may benefit affected children.[184] Conversely, parents may be misinformed regarding the condition,[184] or may have misunderstood the information given.[212,213]

Other research has shown that uptake of antenatal testing is compromised if the test required is invasive. This can also happen if women are not knowledgeable about the test, do not believe it to be reliable or had other anxieties about it, are concerned about miscarriage rates, or if they would not terminate a pregnancy.[213-217] Furthermore, a review of the available research on the psychological effects of antenatal screening concluded that although antenatal diagnosis could provide reassurance for pregnant women, it also created pressures, dilemmas and anxieties.[214] The reviewer argues that the existence of fetal diagnosis means that pregnancy would never again be the same, even for women who decline testing, 'because they will always know that they could have had that knowledge and could have acted on it'.

A survey in Sweden explored the attitudes that influenced women's decisions to accept or decline a serum AFP test.[218] Almost a fifth (19 per cent) of the sample declined, giving anxiety as the reason for their refusal. Many of the women who took the test said that they wanted assurance that the baby was healthy. There were no sociodemographic differences between the women who accepted and those who declined, but religion and attitude towards abortion were significantly different for the two groups. The researchers concluded that it was this rather than the test routine that had a major effect in the decision-making process. Unfortunately, the researchers do not describe what information was available to these women.

An English study of the uptake of screening found that when AFP testing is available, the main factors which influence whether a woman will accept the test include knowledge about the test, attitude to termination and perceived reliability of the test.[219] For amniocentesis the factors include the perceived risks of having an affected child, attitudes to termination and fear of miscarriage. It seems that women having antenatal care are generally underinformed about the tests they are being offered and which they may subsequently undergo. This has been confirmed in other recent work.[184,219,220] It was concluded that if women are to be active participants in decisions about what antenatal tests to undergo, they must be provided with adequate information. This should include the purpose of testing, the condition(s) being screened for, the likelihood that an abnormality will be detected, the test procedures, any risk involved, the meaning of positive and negative test results, and possible actions for a positive result. These include termination, preparing for the birth of a handicapped child and adoption.

These studies have highlighted some of the difficulties faced by both givers and recipients of care in respect of all types of screening tests for genetic conditions. What should be the role of health promotion? Presumably, the aim should be to identify those conditions which have major implications for some or all of the population and which are amenable to intervention, and then to provide information. This should increase the chance that individuals will seek genetic counselling or prenatal screening appropriately.

Should specific sections of the population be the target of health-promotion campaigns about genetic disease, or prenatal screening? These and other questions need to be addressed in evaluative research. In addition, the findings of the Confidential Enquiry into Counselling for Genetic Disorders which is in progress[221] are likely be of relevance to the health-promotion agenda in this area.

Section
4

The first year of life

This section covers a very broad area and we have limited coverage to the topics included in this review. We have not covered interventions aimed at special groups, such as children who have been in a neonatal nursery or in hospital, or children with a disability. Although we have dealt with breastfeeding, advice about weaning and diet in the first year of life has not been covered because of a forthcoming report (during 1994) from the COMA Working Group on Weaning Diet. In addition, an important range of community projects intended to provide social or emotional support for parents has been omitted. Such projects are very diverse in their target populations, their aims and their methods. Evaluations are difficult, though some have been conducted[222,223] and this field has been covered to some extent in other recent reviews.[224]

The arrival of the first baby often changes the relationship between the new parents. Childcare has many practical difficulties and parents, and mothers in particular have to cope with the demands the baby makes upon their physical, emotional, financial and other resources. Parent education aims to prepare people for parenthood by, among other things, providing them with essential information and helping them to develop the skills and problem-solving techniques of parenthood.

Health promotion about baby care is carried out routinely by health visitors, GPs and child health doctors, midwives and others. Books, pamphlets, magazines, newspapers and public and commercial advertising carry all sorts of health-promotion material. Topics include child safety, child development, nutrition, hygiene, immunisation and other aspects of child health surveillance, home care for childhood illnesses and when to seek medical help. The aim is to respond to parents' enquiries and circumstances, and much of it is difficult to describe, far less evaluate. In this part of the report we cover some of the main areas where interventions are likely to have an effect on infant health.

4.1 Interventions to increase the initiation and duration of breastfeeding

Potential impact of health promotion at population level..............................	**Low for serious outcomes, but benefits could apply to all families**
Potential impact of health promotion on individuals	**Low to moderate**
Relevant research	**Extensive, but often methodologically inadequate**
Evidence of impact on behaviour.................	**Low, but suffers from methodological inadequacies**
Evidence of impact on outcomes.................	**Low, but suffers from methodological inadequacies**

Benefits of breastfeeding

Breastfeeding is now generally accepted as being best for babies.[225] The Royal College of Midwives recommend that 'All babies should be exclusively breastfed until they are at least four, and preferably six months old'.[226]

Mature breast milk and its precursor, colostrum (which is produced in the first few days after birth), provide babies with a free, safe, nutritious food which also provides protection against infection.[225,226] Artificial feeds, although probably reasonably safe and nutritious, present problems, which include deficiencies or overabundance of specific essential items such as vitamins. Overconcentrated, overdiluted or contaminated feeds may occur,[227] leading to conditions such as gastroenteritis in the baby.[228] Other benefits of breastfeeding include the mother's own feelings of satisfaction,[229] and the development of the relationship between the mother and her child.[229] On the other hand, there is some evidence from the early postnatal period that breastfeeding may be associated with increased tiredness for mothers,[230] although another study showed that at ten days and three months after birth, mothers who were combining breast and bottle feeding were more tired than either bottle feeders or those fully breastfeeding.[231]

Who breastfeeds?

Table 5 Incidence of breastfeeding in England and Wales 1980, 1985 and 1990. *Source*: OPCS, *Infant Feeding*, 1990.

	1980	1985	1990
No. of women in sample	3755	4671	4942
Percentage who breastfed initially	67	65	64
Percentage of women who were still breastfeeding at 6 weeks	42	40	40

Table 6 Duration of breastfeeding for those who breastfed initially for first and later births (1980, 1985 and 1990, Great Britain). *Source*: OPCS, *Infant Feeding*, 1990

Birth order	Breastfed initially (%)			Breastfed at 6 weeks (%)		
	1980	1985	1990	1980	1985	1990
First births	74	69	69	59	56	57
Later births	58	59	52	67	65	66
All babies	—	—	—	63	61	62

Table 7 Incidence of breastfeeding by mother's age (first birth only) (1980, 1985 and 1990, Great Britain). *Source*: OPCS, *Infant Feeding*, 1990

Mother's age	Breastfed initially (%)		
	1980	1985	1990
Under 20	47	42	39
20–24	69	65	61
25–29	87	81	77
30 or over	86	86	86
All first babies*	74	69	69

* Includes cases where mother's age not known

Table 8 Percentage who breastfed initially by socioeconomic group, as defined by current or last occupation of husband/partner (1980, 1985 and 1990, Great Britain). *Source*: OPCS, *Infant Feeding*, 1990

Socioeconomic group	Breastfed initially (%)		
	1980	1985	1990
I	87	87	86
II	78	81	79
IIINM	77	76	73
All non-manual	80	81	79
IIIM	59	61	59
IV + V	52	54	52
All manual	57	58	57
Unclassified + no partner	52	44	48
All babies	65	64	63

Table 9 Duration of breastfeeding for those who breastfed initially by age at which mother completed full-time education (1980, 1985 and 1990, Great Britain). *Source*: OPCS, *Infant Feeding*, 1990

Age at which mother completed education	Breastfed at 6 weeks (%)		
	1980	1985	1990
16 or under	54	50	52
17 or 18	65	64	63
Over 18	84	81	79
All babies	63	61	62

In England and Wales only 67 per cent of women initially breastfed their babies at least once in 1980 (see Table 5).[53] This decreased marginally to 64 per cent and 65 per cent in 1985 and 1990, respectively.[53] Age, parity, socioeconomic group, education and area of residence are all variables which have been associated with the frequency of breastfeeding (see Tables 6–9).[53]

Factors associated with the continuation of breastfeeding in the 1990 OPCS report included socioeconomic group, education, smoking and alcohol use. Other factors which are known to affect the success or failure of women to initiate and maintain breastfeeding include correct positioning of the baby at the breast, restrictions on the timing and length of feeds, and the effects of combined oestrogen/progesterone contraceptives.[232,233]

Factors which have been shown to be associated with a shorter period of breastfeeding include poor socioeconomic background, the use of drugs in labour, less antenatal education, smoking during pregnancy and a shorter planned duration of breastfeeding.[53]

Research on health-promotion interventions

Health-promotion interventions which have been studied in this field include antenatal information about breastfeeding, the use of specially trained counsellors, not giving free samples of artificial milk, not restricting the length and timing of feeds, not giving supplementary feeds, and teaching mothers to position their babies at the breast.

Strategies for encouraging women to start or to continue to breastfeed

Antenatal education

Antenatal education interventions aimed at encouraging women to breastfeed have been shown to be effective in women of middle to upper socioeconomic status.[234] However, many women who choose to breastfeed appear to do so either before they become pregnant or early in pregnancy, thereby limiting the time available for possible interventions.[235]

Three trials, all American, have examined the giving of information to women in pregnancy.[236-238] Although these trials highlighted the importance of social and psychological influences on breastfeeding decisions, the small unrepresentative samples in the first two studies mean that no generalisations can be made. Furthermore, definitions of what constituted breast- or bottle feeding were not clear. The research methods used were of mixed quality and the method of randomisation was generally not described.

In summary, these trials found that women provided with information about breastfeeding did not necessarily let it affect their choice. Rather, socially acquired attitudes were seen as being more important determinants of the method of feeding chosen, and of the duration of breastfeeding. Improving knowledge without creating positive attitudes about breastfeeding did not increase the incidence or duration of breastfeeding. It seems clear, however, that antenatal education backed up by one-to-one encouragement by a peer counsellor could be efficacious in encouraging women to choose to breastfeed.

The use of lactation counsellors

A number of studies have examined the value of providing postpartum lactation counselling on the duration of breastfeeding.[236-242] Interventions include the provision of a lactation counsellor who instructed the women in the art of 'fixing' the baby to the breast,[239,241] lactation counselling, and telephone contacts[240] and home visits by a counsellor.[242] Again, there were methodological problems with these studies. Trials differed in how breastfeeding was defined, if it was defined at all. Randomisation was not always clearly described and one study used alternate block allocation every two weeks, rather than randomisation.

In summary, the use of lactation counsellors appears to have enhanced women's abilities to maintain breastfeeding for as long as they wanted to, particularly in women from lower socioeconomic groups. Encouragement and support in problem solving was more effective than early initiation of feeding, increased frequency of feeds and discouraging of supplementary feeds.

Free samples of artificial milk

A review of three trials,[243-245] published between 1983 and 1986, of mixed methodological quality, indicated that mothers who were given free samples of artificial milk were more likely to discontinue breastfeeding. On the basis of this work, the review concluded that such free samples should not be given to breastfeeding women.[246] Two other trials[242,247] contribute to the debate on the provision of commercial discharge packs which include free formula samples for breastfeeding mothers. Although again suffering from methodological problems, these studies have also suggested that the provision of artificial milk in discharge packs may provide a risk to the duration of breastfeeding. Providing a breast pump, but no artificial milk, in discharge packs is seen to increase the duration of breastfeeding.

Encouraging early and frequent feeding

One well-designed randomised trial has examined the effects of feeding the baby soon after birth, and not restricting the timing of feeds thereafter.[248] Women who fed their babies within two hours after birth and subsequently whenever they needed, continued to breastfeed for longer and had fewer problems than women who delayed the first feed for four hours and who fed on a fixed schedule.

Positioning the baby at the breast

Ultrasound studies of babies at the breast have demonstrated that pain results from the baby not having a good enough mouthful of breast tissue.[249] This finding has been tested in two randomised controlled trials,[250,251] where it has been shown that women who experience painful nipples when breastfeeding are more likely to continue to breastfeed if they are taught to reposition the baby so that feeding does not hurt. All those working with breastfeeding mothers need to be able to teach this skill.

Policy and breastfeeding

The studies of breastfeeding reviewed so far have pointed to the existence of local policies and practices which did not reflect the findings of research.[252,253] In addition, even where policies are based on evidence, they may be at variance with practice. For example, maternity unit policies which encourage contact between mothers and babies, or breastfeeding soon after delivery, have been observed not to be adhered to in practice.[252] A mismatch between policy and practice has implications for carers, and for mothers and babies.

4.2   Service use in the first year of life

Health promotion aimed at new parents includes information and advice about health-service use. For example, parents are told about the recommended schedule of immunisation and child health surveillance, and they are given information about child health clinics and health visitors. The benefits of immunisation are stressed. Some books include detailed advice about when to seek medical care in the event of childhood illnesses. Taking together health promotion directed at parents and the range of routine systems for offering immunisation and other child health surveillance, the potential for health gain in the total population is probably substantial. There will also be important consequences for individual families, and for the workload of the health service. A recent letter to a paediatric journal[254] highlighted the benefits to an individual family of media publicity about the signs of meningitis.

Although there are studies of the views of parents about general child health services[255,256] and assessments of programmes to encourage immunisation,[257,258] there seem to be few other assessments of health-promotion interventions aimed at increasing the uptake of these services, or encouraging the appropriate use of services. For example, are parent-held child health records being evaluated?

Another important aspect of care in the first year of the child's life is the link between the health of mother and child. Trials have shown that women at risk of postnatal depression can be helped by groups run by a health visitor,[259] and several other studies are in progress or planned which aim to reduce postnatal psychiatric ill-health and improve the outcome for children of women suffering depression. This is an important area for dissemination and further research.

Immunisation

Potential impact of health promotion
   at population level .... **High**
Potential impact of health promotion
   on individual families............................. **High**
Relevant research...................................... **Yes, but difficult to conduct**
Evidence of impact on behaviour................. **Probable**
Evidence of impact on outcomes................. **Probable**

Countries which implement rigorous programmes of immunisation have virtually eliminated many childhood diseases, but when those programmes have been reduced or interrupted epidemics have occurred.[260] In the UK immunisation rates have been increasing for many years. By November 1993, 93 per cent of children had been immunised against diphtheria, tetanus and poliomyelitis by their first birthday, and 91 per cent had been immunised against whooping cough.[261] Uptake of mumps, measles and rubella (MMR) vaccine is also good, with a coverage rate of 92 per cent.[262]

The high level of uptake of immunisation is presumably maintained (or improved) by a combination of direct health promotion to parents, and the systems that make up child health surveillance. No published trials have been discovered which examine the effects of specific health-education programmes on immunisation. With regard to media-driven health-promotion activities, it would be difficult to conduct these types of studies and so the impact of campaigns must be judged by observing the changing patterns of uptake of immunisation and of disease. A recent example is the introduction of immunisation against *haemophilus influenzae* type b (Hib). Prior to the introduction of the vaccine this resulted in 1300 cases of meningitis and 65 deaths each year, mainly in children under 1 year old. When the vaccine was introduced in October 1991, it was estimated that 6 per cent of women with young children had heard of it, and the campaign that followed achieved a striking increase in parents' awareness (73 per cent).[263] At the same time, health professionals were given the relevant information. Coverage has risen to 90 per cent[262] and the it is estimated that the incidence of the disease has dropped by 80 per cent.[257]

Studies on the uptake of childhood immunisation have highlighted the importance of some social factors,[264-266] and there have been some recommendations about targeting advice given by health visitors and GPs. However, different local studies come up with different associations between low uptake and social and attitudinal variables. How should resources be directed to improving uptake in local areas or for specific groups who are reluctant to accept immunisation?

The knowledge and views of care-givers are clearly important. For example, work on pertussis immunisation indicates that in a sample of unimmunised children, 69 per cent (n = 52) had not been immunised, as a result of medical advice.[267] Of these 52 children, 65 per cent were medically advised for reasons which did not conform to the recommended contraindications. Studies of the views of parents make it clear that they need good information from care-givers and time to discuss their concerns.[258,268] A key area for further research in health promotion regarding childhood immunisation is the production and evaluation of information for parents that is sufficiently detailed and easily understood.

4.3   Sudden infant death syndrome

Potential impact of health promotion at population level	**High**
Potential impact of health promotion on individuals	**High**
Relevant research	**Considerable**
Evidence of impact on behaviour	**Probable**
Evidence of impact on outcomes	**Probable**
Evidence of impact on outcomes	**Probable**

Sudden infant death syndrome (SIDS) has been the subject of extensive research but this review coincided with two major and continuing developments. As a result, it was decided that it would be premature to include any detailed review of the topic, for the following reasons. First, after falling very little for over ten years, the post-neonatal mortality rate for England and Wales has started to decline rapidly, from 4.11 per 1000 live births in 1988 to 2.30 in 1992. Although this fall can be seen in most causes of death, those attributed to SIDS have made a major contribution to the fall. The rate of post-neonatal deaths certified as 'sudden infant death,' or where cot death or a similar term was mentioned on the certificate, decreased from 2.18 per 1000 in 1988 to 1.35 per 1000 in 1991. Corresponding figures for 1992 have yet to be published, but the total number of deaths in children under 15 coded to ICD 798.0 fell from 1050 in 1991 to 456 in 1992. The relative contributions of the various factors, including advice to parents about sleeping position, that could have produced this striking fall are currently under investigation.

In addition, the report of the Chief Medical Officer's Expert Group on the sleeping position of infants and cot death was published just as this review was being completed. It concluded that there were causal relationships between sleeping in the prone position and increased numbers of cot deaths. There were also strong relationships between mothers smoking and cot deaths. Furthermore, babies suffering a cot death were seen to have been at greater risk of overheating.[269]

The Expert Group recommended that babies should not be laid to sleep on their fronts, except in particular circumstances on medical advice, and that the great majority should be put on their backs; that babies should not be exposed to cigarette smoke either before birth or afterwards; and that babies should not be overwrapped or overheated, especially when they are feverish or unwell.[269]

Finally, a marginally different category of 'sudden unexpected death' has been chosen for special investigation in the Confidential Enquiry into Stillbirths and Deaths in Infancy, which is now under way.

4.4 Accidental injury

Accidental injury is a major cause of fatal and non-fatal injury in the under-fives.[8] It has been identified in *The Health of the Nation* as a key area for improvement. The target is for mortality due to childhood accidents to be reduced from 6.6 per 100,000 head of population in 1990 to 4.4 per 100,000 by the year 2005. Research on accidental injury in childhood is the topic of a recent Health Education Authority review.[45] The reviewers examined health-promotion interventions aimed at preventing childhood accidents among children aged 0–14 years in the home, at leisure areas – for example in playgrounds, swimming areas and so on – and on the roads. The number of children under the age of 1 who have accidental injuries is small.

There are few evaluated studies on accidental injury, and only a limited number of interventions available.[45] Furthermore, some types of accident prevention were more researched, for example the effect of car safety restraints for children. Single-measure interventions, such as window bars in the home and car child safety restraints, were particularly effective because they had a single focus. The success of campaigns was increased by improving availability and reducing the costs of the measures. Some injury types, such as scalds and other home injuries, cannot be addressed by single-measure strategies, and health-promotion campaigns have met with limited success.[45] Community-based programmes have positive results but take longer to become effective, as alliances need to develop between individuals, policy makers and the communities. This is an area where direct health promotion to parents is only part of a complex set of strategies involving planners, manufacturers, those who set product standards and a range of health policy makers and care-givers. For babies, the key areas for action are probably car-seat schemes and some aspects of home safety, such as child proof containers and fireguards. In the UK on hospital discharge most babies still sit on their mother's knee in the rear of the car. Evaluations of child car restraint loan schemes show modest benefits in terms of correct use.[270] Campaigns about home safety aimed at parents have had mixed results.[45]

4.5   Non-accidental injury

Non-accidental injury and neglect are important causes of childhood injuries and make an appreciable contribution to childhood mortality.[271] Multidisciplinary care involving the paediatric, nursing, psychiatric and legal professions is required for these children and their families. Multidisciplinary research has made it possible to decide how to give care using earlier diagnosis and more successful treatment programmes.[272]

Although it is not possible to discuss child abuse and neglect in any detail here, it will briefly be noted that observational studies have suggested that early and extended postpartum support at home improves mothers' attachment to their babies.[272] It is not clear from this study whether there is an associated decrease in child abuse and neglect. Other work has suggested that women may show the same amount of 'abnormal parenting behaviours', even after the treatment group was included in an intervention programme to improve their parenting skills. However, the injury to the child showed a qualitative difference: children of parents in the treatment group did not require hospitalisation, that is, they may have had cigarette burns or scratches, for example, rather than broken bones and head injuries.[271]

Reports of serious child abuse have become all too frequent in the media. The ultimate aim of health promotion would be to prevent any form of non-accidental injury to children. Although it is difficult to conduct trials that look at the efficacy of educational programmes for people who abuse or neglect their children, research which examines their motivation could provide the type of information needed for the development of self-help behavioural strategies. The efficacy of these strategies could then be monitored and assessed.

Section
5

Recommendations for research

- The most promising behavioural interventions for stopping smoking should be tested in the UK in methodologically sound controlled trials based on normal health service provision.

- Future trials of anti-smoking interventions could, in addition to smoking cessation rates, include as outcomes longer-term abstinence, in particular postnatal abstinence; main perinatal health outcomes; infant health outcomes; maternal psychosocial outcomes; and maternal health outcomes.

- Further research is needed on effective and cost-effective ways of identifying and helping pregnant women who consume too much alcohol.

- Research about diet and parenthood should seek to unravel some of the complex interactions with other social factors and explore ways of improving health outcomes for subgroups of the population about whom there is particular concern.

- Research is needed to evaluate direct health promotion to prospective parents about dietary supplementation aimed at reducing the risk of neural tube defects.

- Further research is needed in order to give women and care-givers far clearer guidance about the positive and negative effects of physical effort at home, in the workplace and in recreation. Health promotion on these topics will be of increased value once the necessary research information is available.

- The benefits of genetic counselling on populations, individuals and families have not been subject to evaluation. Research that looks at what counselling is provided and its effects on reproductive decision making is needed. Where parents choose to have an affected child, research should focus on interventions that aim to help the family cope.

- Reviews of health promotion aimed at improving the physical and mental health of recent mothers would be of value.

● Reviews of health promotion directed at 'softer' outcomes in pregnancy and parenthood would complement this review. In particular, community projects aimed at supporting parents are potentially important and have not been reviewed.

● Systematic reviewing of studies of health-promotion interventions can be carried out in different ways, which may yield different conclusions. There is a need for wider debate about the methods of reviewing, and an awareness of the methodological issues involved in judging the usefulness of research studies.

● A key area for further research in health promotion in relation to childhood immunisation is the production and evaluation of information for parents that is sufficiently detailed and easily understood.

Bibliography

1 Department of Health (1990) *Confidential enquiry into stillbirths and deaths in infancy.* London, HMSO.

2 Department of Health (1992) *Health of the nation: a strategy for health in England.* London, HMSO.

3 Roussounis, S.H., Hubley, P.A. and Dear, P.R.F. (1993) 'Five-year-follow-up of very low birth-weight infants: neurological and physiological outcome', *Child Care Health and Development.* vol 19, pp.45-59.

4 Griffin, J. (1993) *Born too soon.* Office of Health Economics, London.

5 Hein, H.A., Burmeister, L.F. and Papke, K.R. (1990) 'The relationship of unwed status to infant mortality'. *Obstetrics and Gynecology*, vol 76, pp.763-8.

6 Rice, N.C. and Friedman, E. (1987) 'A model for training health professionals in disease prevention and health promotion', in *Proceedings of the 12th World Conference on Health Education*, Dublin, 1–6 September 1985.

7 Short, R. (1980) *Second report from the Social Services Committee, perinatal and neonatal mortality.* House of Commons Paper, 663–1 (Session 1979-80), HMSO, London.

8 Office of Population Censuses and Surveys (published annually) *Mortality statistics - perinatal and infant: social and biological factors.* Series DH3, HMSO, London.

9 Macfarlane, A. and Mugford, M. (1984) *Birth counts: statistics of pregnancy and childbirth.* 2 volumes. HMSO, London.

10 Alberman, E. (1992) *Memorandum to House of Commons Health Committee on Maternity Services*, vol II, HC 29 -II. HMSO, London.

11 Parsons, L., Macfarlane, A. and Golding, J. (1993) 'Pregnancy, birth and maternity care' in Ahmad, W. (ed.) *'Race' and health in contemporary Britain.* Open University Press, Milton Keynes, pp.51-75.

12 Balajaran, R. and McDowall, M. (1985) 'Mortality from congenital malformations by mother's country of birth', *Journal of Epidemiology and Community Health.* vol 39, pp.102-6.

13 Balajaran, R., Raleigh, V.S. and Botting, B. (1989) 'Mortality from congenital malformations in England and Wales: variations by mother's country of birth', *Archives of Diseases in Child-hood.* vol 64, pp.1457-62.

14 Balajaran, R. and Botting, B. (1989) 'Perinatal mortality in England and Wales: variations by mother's country of birth (1982-85)', *Health Trends.* vol 21, pp.79-84.

15 Balajaran, R. and Raleigh, V.S. (1993) 'The ethnic populations of England and Wales: the 1991 census', *Health Trends.* vol 24, pp.113-16.

16 Libbus, M.K. and Sable, M.R. (1991) 'Prenatal education in a high risk population: the effects on birth outcomes', *Birth.* vol 18, no.2, pp.78-82.

17 Papiernik, E., Bouyer, J. Dreyfus, J. *et al.* (1985) 'Prevention of preterm births: a perinatal study in Haguenau, France, *Pediatrics.* vol 76, pp.154-8.

18 Institute of Medicine, Committee to Study the Prevention of Low Birthweight, Division of Health promotion and Disease Prevention (1985). *Preventing low birthweight.* National Academy Press, Washington.

19 Main, D.M., Gabbe, S.G., Richardson, D. and Strong, S. (1985) 'Can preterm deliveries be prevented?' *American Journal Obstetrics and Gynecology*, vol 151. pp.892-8.

20 Leon, Da., Vagero, D. and Olausson, P.O. (1992) 'Social class differences in infant mortality in Sweden: comparison with England and Wales', *British Medical Journal.* vol 305, pp.687-91.

21 Heins, H.C., Nance, N.W., McCarthy, B.J. and Efird, C.M. (1990) 'A randomised trial of nurse-midwifery prenatal care to reduce low birth-weight', *Obstetrics and Gynecology*. vol 75, pp.341–5.

22 Hobel, C.J. and Bemis, R.L. (1986) The West Area Los Angeles Prematurity Prevention Demonstration Project, in: Papiernik, E., Breart, G. and Spira, N. (eds.) *Prevention of preterm birth*. INSERM, vol 138, pp.205–22.

23 OPCS Monitor (1993), DH3 93/2, Sept 1993. HMSO, London.

24 Royal College of Physicians (1989). *Prenatal diagnosis and genetic screening; community and service implications*. RCP, London.

25 Sarjeant, G.R. (1985) *Sickle cell disease*. Oxford University Press, Oxford.

26 Weatherall D. J. and Clegg, J.B. (1984) *The thalassaemia syndromes*. Blackwell Scientific Publications, Oxford.

27 Whitehead, M. and Tones, K. (1991) *Avoiding the pitfalls: notes on the planning and implementation of health education strategies and the special role of the Health Education Authority*. HEA, London.

28 Combes, G. and Schonveld, A. 1992 *Life will never be the same again – learning to be a first-time parent: a review of antenatal and post-natal health education*. HEA, London.

29 Expert Maternity Group (1993). *Changing childbirth*. HMSO, London.

30 Curtice, L. (1989) *The first year of life: promoting the health of babies in the community*. Maternity Alliance, London.

31 Health Education Authority (1993). *The new pregnancy book (1993/4): a complete guide to pregnancy, childbirth and the first few weeks with a new baby*. HEA, London.

32 Bounty (1989). *The Bounty mother-to-be book*. Bounty Publications.

33 Bounty (1990). *Parentcraft: the class textbook*. Bounty Publications.

34 Health Education Authority (1991). *Birth to five: a guide to the first five years of being a parent*. HEA, London.

35 Health Education Authority (1992). *Childhood diseases haven't died. Children have*. also *MMR and Hib immunisation*. 3 leaflets, HEA, London. 1992.

36 Health Education Authority (1992). *Breast-feeding. Your questions answered by the Health Education Authority*. HEA, London.

37 Health Education Authority (1991). *From milk to mixed feeding*. HEA, London.

38 Health Education Authority (1992). *Maternal and child health clinics*. HEA, London.

39 National Dairy Council (1987). *A guide for the expectant mother*. NDC, London.

40 Wyeth Nutrition. *Breastfeeding your baby*. Leaflet.

41 NALGO. *Maternity and caring rights*. A NALGO negotiating guide.

42 Peaudouce. *Life after baby; a Peaudouce guide to post-natal problems*. Leaflet.

43 Child Accident Prevention Trust (1990/91). *Keep them safe: a guide to child safety equipment*, and *Keep your baby safe: a guide to safe nursery equipment*. Leaflets.

44 Hodnett E. (1993) 'Support from care-givers during childbirth,' in Enkin, M.W., Keirse, M.J.N.C., Renfrew, M.J., Neilson, J.P. (eds.) *Pregnancy and childbirth module*. Review No. 03871, Cochrane Database of Systematic Reviews, Cochrane Updates on Disk, Oxford, Update Software.

45 Towner, E., Dowswell, T. and Jarvis, S. (1993) *Reducing childhood accidents – the effectiveness of health promotion interventions: a literature review*. HEA, London.

46 Marsh, A. and Matheson J. (1983) *Smoking attitudes and behaviour*. HMSO, OPCS, London.

47 World Health Organization (1985). *Evaluation of the carcinogenic risks of chemicals to humans: tobacco smoking*. International Agency for Research on Cancer, Monograph 38.

48 Kleinmann, J.C. and Madans, J.H. (1985) 'The effects of maternal smoking, physical stature and educational attainment on the incidence on low birthweight'. *American Journal of Epidemiology*. vol 121, no.6, pp.843–54.

49 Burchfiel, C.M., Higgins, M.W., Keller, J.B., Howatt, W.F., Butler, W.J. and Higging, I.T.T. (1986) 'Passive smoking and pulmonary function

in Tecumseh, Michigan', *American Review of Respiratory Diseases*. vol 133, no.6, pp.966-73.

50 Bellinger, D., Leviton, A., Needleman, H.L., Waternaux, C. and Rabinowitz, M. (1986) 'Low-level lead exposure and infant development in the first year', *Neurobehavior, Toxicology and Teratology*, vol 8, no.2, pp.151-61.

51 Bonithon-Kopp., C., Huel, G., Moreau, T. and Wending, R. (1986) 'Prenatal exposure to lead and cadmium and psychomotor development of the child at 6 years', *Neurobehavior Toxicology Teratology*, vol 8, no.3, pp.307-10.

52 Office of Population Censuses and Surveys (1992). *General Household Survey 1990. An inter-departmental survey carried out by OPCS between April 1990 and March 1991*. HMSO, London.

53 White, A., Freeth, S. and O'Brien M. (1990) *Infant Feeding*. OPCS, HMSO, London.

54 Graham, H. (1992) *Smoking among working class mothers: final report*. Department of Applied Social Studies, University of Warwick.

55 Action on Smoking and Health (1993). *Her share of misfortune - women, smoking and low income*. Derry, Nottingham.

56 Walsh, R and Redman, S. (1993) 'Smoking cessation in pregnancy: do effective programmes exist?', *Health Promotion International*, vol 8, pp.111-27.

57 Lumley, J. (1993) 'Strategies for reducing smoking in pregnancy', in Enkin, M.W., Keirse, M.J.N.C., Renfrew, M.J. and Neilson, J.P. (eds.) *Pregnancy and childbirth module*, Review No. 03312 Cochrane Database of Systematic Reviews, Cochrane Updates on Disk, Oxford, Update Software.

58 Health Education Authority (1994). *Smoking and pregnancy: guidance for purchasers and providers*. HEA, London.

59 Loeb, B.K., Waage, G. and Bailey, J. (1983) Smoking intervention in pregnancy. *Proceedings of 5th World Conference on Smoking and Health, Winnipeg*, vol 1, pp.389-395.

60 Bauman, K.E., Bryan, E.S., Dent, C.W. and Koch, G.G. (1983) 'The influence of observing carbon monoxide level on cigarette smoking by public prenatal patients', American Journal of Public Health', vol 73, pp.1089-91.

61 Power, F.L., Gillies, P.A., Madeley, R.J. and Abbott, M. (1989) 'Research in an antenatal clinic - the experience of the Nottingham Mothers' Stop Smoking Project', *Midwifery*, vol 5, pp.106-12.

62 Reading, A.E., Campbell, S., Cox, D.N. and Sledmore, C.M. (1982) 'Health beliefs and health care behaviour in pregnancy', *Psychological Medicine*, vol 12, pp.379-83.

63 Graham, H. (1987) 'Women's smoking and family health', *Social Science and Medicine*, vol 25, no.1, pp.47-56.

64 Jones, K. and MacLeod-Clarke, J. (1993) 'Smoking and pregnancy: the role of health professionals', *Health Visitor*. vol 66, no.3, 1993, pp.88-90.

65 Graham, H. (1976) 'Smoking in pregnancy: the attitudes of expectant mothers', *Social Science and Medicine*. vol 10, pp.399-405.

66 Kokotailo, P.K., Adger, H. Jr, Duggan, A.K., Repke, J. and Joffe, A. (1992) 'Cigarette, alcohol and other drug use by school-age pregnant adolescents: prevalence, detection and associated risk factors', *Pediatrics*. vol 90, no.3, pp.328-34.

67 American Journal of Public Health (1993) 'Effects of in-utero exposure to street drugs', *American Journal of Public Health*, Suppl, vol 83.

68 Cherukuri, R., Minkoff, H., Feldman, J., Parekh, A. and Glass, L. (1988) 'A cohort study of alkaloidal cocaine ('crack') in pregnancy', *Obstetrics and Gynecology*, vol. 72, pp.147-51.

69 MacGregor, S.N., Keith, L.G., Bachicha, J.A. and Chasnoff, I.J. (1989) 'Cocaine abuse during pregnancy: correlation between prenatal care and perinatal outcome', *Obstetrics and Gynecology*, vol 74, pp.882-5.

70 Critchley, H.O., Woods, S.M., Barson, A.J., Richardson, T. and Liberman, B.A. (1988) 'Fetal death in utero and cocaine abuse: a case report', *British Journal of Obstetrics and Gynecology*. vol 95, pp.195-6.

71 Zuckerman, B.S., Frank, D.A., Hingson, R. (1989) 'The effects of maternal marijuana and cocaine use on fetal growth', *New England Journal of Medicine*. vol 320, pp.762-8.

72 Bauchner, H., Zuckerman, B., McClain, M., Frank, D.A., Fired, L.E. and Kayne, H. (1988) 'Risk of sudden infant death syndrome among infants with in utero exposure to cocaine'. *Journal of Pediatrics*. vol 113, pp.831-4.

73 McDonnell, R. and Maynard, A. (1985) 'Estimation of life years lost from alcohol related premature death',. *Alcohol and Alcoholism*, vol 20, pp.435-43.

74 Health Education Authority (1993) *Health Update No. 3, Alcohol.* HEA, London.

75 Nuffield Institute for Health, University of Leeds, Centre for Health Economics, University of York, Research Unit, Royal College of Physicians (1993) 'Brief interventions and alcohol use.' *Effective Health Care.* No7, November.

76 Stein, Z. and Kline, J. (1983) 'Smoking, alcohol and reproduction', *American Journal of Public Health*. vol 73, pp.1154-56.

77 Waterson, E.J. and Murray-Lyon, I.M. (1990) 'Preventing alcohol related birth damage: a review', *Social Science and Medicine*. vol 30, no.3), pp.349-64.

78 EUROMAC Project Group (1992) 'EUROMAC: Maternal alcohol consumption and its relation to the outcome of pregnancy and child development at 18 months', *International Journal of Epidemiology*, vol 21, Suppl.1.

79 Plant, M. (1985) *Women, drinking and pregnancy.* Tavistock, London.

80 Hawkes, S.R. (1993) 'Fetal alcohol syndrome: implications for health education', *Journal of Health Education*. vol 24 no.1, pp.22-6.

81 Plant, M. (1985) 'Fetal alcohol syndrome: an overview', *Midwifery*. vol 1, pp.225-31.

82 Breeze, E. (1984) *Women and drinking*. HMSO, OPCS, London.

83 Masis, K.B. and May, P.A. (1991) 'A comprehensive local program for the prevention of fetal alcohol syndrome', *Public Health Reports*. vol 106, no.5, pp.484-9.

84 Waterson, E.J. and Murray-Lyon, I.M. (1988) 'Asking about alcohol: a comparison of three methods used in an antenatal clinic', *Journal of Obstetrics and Gynaecology*. vol 8, pp.303-6.

85 Ihlen, B.M., Amundsen, A. and Tronnes, L. (1993) 'Reduced alcohol use in pregnancy and changed attitudes in the population', *Addiction*. vol 88, pp.389-94.

86 Waterson, E.J. and Murray-Lyon, I.M. (1990) 'Preventing fetal alcohol effects: a trial of three methods of giving information in the antenatal clinic', *Health Education Research*. vol 5, no.1, pp. 53-61.

87 Brief interventions and alcohol use. *Effective Health Care*, No7, Nov 1993.

88 Paul, A.A., Muller, E.M., and Whitehead, R.G. (1973) 'The quantitative effects of maternal dietary energy intake on pregnancy and lactation in rural Gambian women', *Transactions of the Royal Society of Tropical Medicine and Hygiene*. vol 73, pp.686-92.

89 Ebbs, J.H., Scott, W.A., Tisdall, F.F., Moyle, W.J. and Bell M. (1942) 'Nutrition in pregnancy', *Canadian Medical Association Journal*. vol 46, pp.1-6.

90 Smith, C.A. (1947) 'Effects of maternal under-nutrition upon the newborn infant in Holland (1944-1945)', *Journal of Pediatrics*. vol 30, p.229.

91 Anatonov, A.N. (1947) 'Children born during the siege of Leningrad in 1942', *Journal of Pediatrics*. vol 30, p.250.

92 Gruenwald, P. and Funakawa, I.L. (1967) 'Influence of environmental factors on fetal growth in man', *Lancet*. vol 1, p.1026.

93 Institute of Medicine (1990) *Nutrition during pregnancy: weight gain and nutrition supplementation*. National Academy Press, Washington DC.

94 Rush, D., Alvir, J.M., Kenny, D.A., Johnson, S.S. and Horwitz, D.G. (1988) 'Historical study of pregnancy outcomes in the national WIC evaluation. Evaluation of Special Supplemental Food Programme for Women, Infants and Children', *American Journal of Clinical Nutrition.*, vol 48, pp.412-28.

95 Kramer, M.S. (1993) 'Effects of energy and protein intakes on pregnancy outcome: an overview of the research evidence from controlled clinical trials', *American Journal of Clinical Nutrition*. vol 58, pp.627-35.

96 Hunt, I.F., Jacob, M., Ostergard, N.J., Masri, G., Clark, V.A. and Coulson, A.H. (1976) 'Effect of nutrition education on the nutritional status of low income pregnant women of Mexican descent', *American Journal of Clinical Nutrition*, vol 29, pp.675–84.

97 Zeskind, P.S. and Ramey, C.T. (1981) 'Preventing intellectual and interactional sequelae of fetal malnutrition: a longitudinal, transactional and synergistic app.roach to development', *Child Development*, vol 52, pp.213–18.

98 Barker, D.J.P., Gluckman, P.D., Godfrey, K.M., and Harding, J.E. (1993) 'Fetal nutrition and cardiovascular disease in later life', *Lancet*, vol 341, pp.938–41.

99 Barker, D.J.P., Martyn, C.N., Osmond, C., Hales, C.N. (1993) 'Growth in utero and serum cholesterol concentrations in adult life', *British Medical Journal*, vol 307, pp.1524–7.

100 Durnin, J.V.G.A. (1987) 'Energy requirements of pregnancy: an integration of the longitudinal data from the five country study', *Lancet*. vol ii, pp.1131–3.

101 Van Raaij, J.A.T.M., Vermatt-Miedema, S.H., Schonk, C.M., Peck, P.E.M. and Hautvast, J.G.A.G. (1987) 'Energy requirements in pregnancy in the Netherlands', *Lancet*. vol ii, pp.953–4.

102 Department of Health (1991) *Dietary reference values for food energy and nutrients for the United Kingdom*. Report on Health and Social Subjects, No.41, HMSO, London.

103 Rosa, F.W., Wilk, A.L. and Kelsey, F.O. (1986) 'Teratogen update: vitamin A congeners', *Teratology*. vol 33, pp.355–64.

104 Teratology Society (1987) 'Recommendations for vitamin A use during pregnancy', *Teratology*. vol 35, pp.269–75.

105 Department of Health (1990) *Women cautioned: watch your vitamin A intake*. Department of Health, London.

106 Chanarin, J. (1979) *The megaloblastic anaemias*. 2nd Edn. Blackwell Scientific, Oxford.

107 Mahomed, K. (1993) 'Routine folate supplementation in pregnancy', in Enkin, M.W., Keirse, M.J.N.C., Renfrew, M.J. and Neilson, J.P. (eds.) *Pregnancy and childbirth module*. Review No.

03158, Cochrane Database of Systematic Reviews, Cochrane Updates on Disk, Oxford, Update Software.

108 Lumley, J. (1993) 'Periconceptional folate (4 mg/day) vs placebo in high-risk mothers', in Enkin, M.W., Keirse, M.J.N.C., Renfrew, M.J. and Neilson, J.P. (eds.) *Pregnancy and childbirth module*, Review No. 06488, Cochrane Database of Systematic Reviews, Cochrane Updates on Disk, Oxford, Update Software.

109 Medical Research Council Vitamin Study Research Group (1991). 'Prevention of neural tube defects: results of the Medical Research Council vitamin study', *Lancet*. vol 338, pp.131–7.

110 Lumley, J. (1993) 'Periconceptual multivitamins (incl folate 0.8 mg) vs placebo', in Enkin, M.W., Keirse, M.J.N.C., Renfrew, M.J. and Neilson, J.P. (eds.) *Pregnancy and childbirth module*. Review No. 06490, Cochrane Database of Systematic Reviews, Cochrane Updates on Disk, Oxford, Update Software.

111 Werler, M.M., Shapiro, S. and Mitchell, A.A. (1993) 'Periconceptual folic acid exposure and risk of occurent neural tube defects', *Journal of the American Medical Association*. vol 269, no.10, pp.1257–61.

112 Czeizel, A.E. and Dudas, I. (1992) 'Prevention of first occurrence of neural tube defects by periconceptual vitamin supplementation'. *New England journal of Medicine*. vol 327, no.26, pp.1832–5.

113 Department of Health. (1992) *Folic acid and the prevention of neural tube defects: Report from an Expert Advisory Group*. Health Publications Unit, Lancashire.

114 Editorial (1993) 'Folic acid-preventable spina bifida and anencephaly'. *Journal of the American Medical Association*. vol 269, no.10, pp.1292–3.

115 Centers for Disease Control and Prevention (1992) 'Recommendations for the use of folic acid to reduce the number of cases of spina bifida and other neural tube defects', *Mortality Morbidity Weekly Reports*, vol 41, No.R-R-14, pp.1233–8.

116 Alleva, F.R., Alleva, J.J. and Balzs, T. (1976) 'Effect of large daily doses of ascorbic acid on pregnancy in guinea pig, rats and hamsters', *Toxicology and Applied Pharmacology*. vol 35, pp.393–5.

117 Cockburn, F., Belton, N.R. and Purvis, R.J. (1980) 'Maternal vitamin D intake and mineral metabolism in mothers and their new-born infants', *British Medical Journal*. vol 281, pp.11–14.

118 Purdie, D.W. (1989) 'Bone mineral metabolism and reproduction'. *Contemporary Reviews in Obstetrics and Gynaecology*, vol 1, pp.214–21.

119 Chan, G.M., McMurray, M., Westover, K., Englebert-Fenton, K. and Thomas, M.R. (1987) 'Effects of increased dietary calcium and bone mineral status in lactating adolescent and adult women', *American Journal of Clinical Nutrition*. vol 46, pp.319–23.

120 Lumley, J. (1993) 'Routine calcum supplementation in pregnancy', in Enkin, M.W., Keirse, M.J.N.C., Renfrew, M.J. and Neilson, J.P. (eds.) *Pregnancy and childbirth module*. Review No. 05938, Cochrane Database of Systematic Reviews, Cochrane Updates on Disk, Oxford, Update Software.

121 Mahomed, K. (1993) 'Routine iron supplementation in pregnancy', in Enkin, M.W., Keirse, M.J.N.C., Renfrew, M.J. and Neilson, J.P. (eds.) *Pregnancy and childbirth module*. Review No. 03157, Cochrane Database of Systematic Reviews, Cochrane Updates on Disk, Oxford, Update Software.

122 Durward, L. (1988) *Poverty in pregnancy: the cost of an adequate diet for expectant mothers*. Maternity Alliance, London.

123 Doyle, W., Crawford, M.A., Laurance, B.M. and Drury, P. (1982) 'Dietary survey in pregnancy in a low socio-economic group', *Human Nutrition: Applied Nutrition*, vol 36A, pp.95–106.

124 Doyle, W., Crawford, M.A., Wynn, A.H.A. and Wynn, S.W. (1989) 'Maternal nutrient intake and birthweight', *Journal of Human Nutrition and Diet*. vol 2, pp.415–22.

125 Nelson, M. (1990) 'Vitamin A and risk of birth defects', *British Medical Journal*. vol 301, pp.1176.

126 McKnight, A. and Merrett, D. (1981) 'Nutriton in pregnancy – a health education problem', *Practitioner*. vol 231, no.1427, pp.530–8.

127 Endres, J.M., Poell-Odenwald, K., Sawicki, M. and Welch, P. (1985) 'Dietary assessment of pregnant adolescents participating in a supplemental food programme', *Journal of Reproductive Medicine*. vol 30, no.1, pp.10–17.

128 Ancri, G., Morse, E.H. and Clarke, R.P. (1977) 'Comparison of the nutritional status of pregnant adolescents with adult pregnant women. III Maternal protein and calorie intake and weight gain in relation to size at infant birth'. *American Journal of Clinical Nutrition*. vol 30, pp.568–72.

129 Kaminetsky, H.A., Langer, A. and Baker, H. (1973) 'The effect of nutrition in teenage gravidas on pregnancy and the state of the neonate. I. A nutritional profile', *American Journal of Obstetrics and Gynecology*. vol 115, pp.639–46.

130 American Dietetic Association (1989) 'Position of the American Dietetic Association: nutrition management in adolescent pregnancy', *Journal of the American Dietetic Association*. vol 89, pp.104–9.

131 Frisancho, A.R., Matos, J., Leonard, W.R. and Allen Yaroch, L. (1985) 'Developmental and nutritional determinants of pregnancy outcome among teenagers', *American Journal of Physical Anthropology*. vol 66, No.3, pp.247–61.

132 Scholl, T.O., Hediger, M.L. and Ances, I.G. (1990) Maternal growth during pregnancy and decreased infant birth weight,' *American Journal of Clinical Nutrition*. vol 51, pp.790–3.

133 Stevens-Simon, C. and McAnarney, E.R. (1988) 'Adolescent maternal weight gain and low birth weight: a multifactorial model', *American Journal of Clinical Nutrition*. vol 47, pp.948–53.

134 McFadyen, I.R., Campbell-Brown, M., Abraham, R., North, W.R.S. and Haines, A.P. (1984) 'Factors affecting birthweight in Hindus, Moslems and Europeans', *British Journal of Obstetrics and Gynecology*. vol 91, pp.968–72.

135 Clarson, C.L., Barter, M.J., Marshall, T. and Wharton, B.A. (1982) 'Secular changes in birthweight of Asian babies born in Birmingham', *Archives of Diseases in Childhood*. vol 57, pp. 867–71.

136 Eaton, P.M., Wharton, P.A. and Wharton, B.A. (1984) 'Nutrient intake of pregnant Asian women at Sorrento Maternity Hospital Birmingham', *British Journal of Nutrition.* vol 52, no.3, pp.457–68.

137 Abraham, R., Campbell-Brown, M., North, W.R.S. and McFadyen, I.R. (1987) 'Diets of Asian pregnant women in Harrow: iron and vitamins'. *Human Nutrition Applied Nutrition.* vol 41A, pp.164–73.

138 Wharton, P.A., Eaton, P.M. and Wharton, B.A. (1984) 'Subethnic variation in the diets of Moslem, Sikh and Hindu pregnant women at Sorrento Maternity Hospital, Birmingham', *British Journal of Nutrition.* vol 52, no.3, pp.469–76.

139 Reeves, J. (1992) 'Pregnancy and fasting during Ramadan', (Letter), *British Medical Journal.* vol 304, pp.843–4.

140 Brozovic, M. (1992) 'Sickle cell disease', *Prescribers' Journal.* vol 32, no.2, pp.45–55.

141 Allen, C.D. and Ries, C.P. (1985) 'Smoking, alcohol and dietary practices during pregnancy: comparison before and after prenatal education', *Journal of the American Dietetic Association.* vol 85, no.5, pp.605–6.

142 Daelhousen, B.B. and Guthrie, H.A. (1982) 'A self-instruction program for pregnant women', *Journal of the American Dietetic Association.* vol 81, no.4, pp.407–412.

143 Perkin, J. (1983) Evaluating a nutrition education programme for pregnant teenagers: cognitive vs behavioral outcomes', *Journal of School Health.* vol 53, no.7, pp.420–22.

144 Anderson, A.S. and Shepherd, R. (1989) 'Beliefs and attitudes toward 'healthier eating' among women attending maternity hospital', *Journal of Nutrition Education,* vol 21, no.5, pp.208–213.

145 Kafatos, A.G., Vlachonicholis, I.G. and Codrington, C.A. (1989) 'Nutrition during pregnancy: the effects of an educational intervention programme in Greece', *American Journal of Clinical Nutrition.* vol 50, pp.970–9.

146 Orstead, C., Arrington, D., Kamath, S.K., Olson, R. and Kohrs, M.B. (1985) 'Efficacy of prenatal nutrition counselling: weightgain, infant birthweight and cost effectiveness', *Journal of American Dietetic Association.* vol 85, no.1, pp.40–5.

147 Association of Medical Microbiologists (1989) *The facts about listeria.* AMM, London.

148 Department of Health (1992) *Management and prevention of listeriosis and other food borne infections in pregnancy.* PL/CMO (92) 19, PL/CNO (92) 13, London.

149 Redman, C. and Walker, I. (1992) *Pre-eclampsia - the facts.* Oxford University Press, Oxford.

150 Green, J. (1989) 'Diet and the prevention of pre-eclampsia,' in Chalmers, I., Enkin, M. and Keirse, M.J.N.C. (eds.) *Effective care in pregnancy and childbirth,* Oxford University Press, Oxford.

151 Hankin, M.E. and Symonds, E.M. (1962) 'Body weight, diet and pre-eclamptic toxaemia in pregnancy', *Australia and New Zealand Journal of Obstetrics and Gynecology.* vol 4, pp.156–60.

152 Jelsema, R.D., Bhatia, R.K. Zador, I.E., Bottoms, S.F. and Sokol, R.J. (1991) 'Is placenta previa a determinant of preeclampsia?', *Journal of Perinatal Medicine.* vol 19, pp.485–8.

153 Wallenburg, H.C.S., Dekker, G.A., Markovitz, J.W. and Rotmans, P. (1986) 'Low-dose aspirin prevents pregnancy-induced hypertension and preeclampsia in angiotensin-sensitive primigravidae', *Lancet.* vol i, pp.1–3.

154 Smith, C.A. (1947) 'The effect of wartime starvation in Holland upon pregnancy and its product', *American Journal of Obstetrics and Gynecology.* vol 53, pp.599–606.

155 Miles, J.F., Martin, J.N., Blake, P.G., Perry, K.G., Martin, R.W. and Meeks, G.R.(1990) 'Postpartum eclampsia: a recurring perinatal dilemma', *Obstetrics and Gynecology.* vol 76, no.3, pp.328–31.

156 Naeye, R.L. and Peters, E.C. (1982) 'Working during pregnancy: effects on the fetus', *Pediatrics.* vol 66, pp.724–72.

157 Zuckerman, B.S., Frank, D.A., Hingson, R. *et al.* (1986) 'Impact of maternal work outside the home during pregnancy on neonatal outcome', *Pediatrics.* vol 77, pp.459–64.

158 Peters, T.J., Adelstein, P., Golding, J. and Butler, N.R. (1984) 'The effects of work in pregnancy: short- and long-term associations' in Chamberlain, G. (ed.) *Pregnant women at work.* Royal Society of Medicine, London, pp.87–104.

159 Garcia, J. and Elbourne, D.E. (1984) 'Future research on work and pregnancy', in Chamberlain, G. (ed.) *Pregnant women at work*, Royal Society of Medicine, London, pp.273-87.

160 Saurel-Cubizolles, M-J. and Kaminski, M. (1990) 'Is preterm delivery rate still associated with physical working conditions?' *Journal of Epidemiology and Community Health*. vol 45, pp.29-34.

161 Mamelle, N., Laumon, B. and Lazar, P. (1984) 'Prematurity and occupational activity during pregnancy'. *American Journal of Epidemiology*. vol 119, p.30.

162 Mamelle, N. and Laumon, B. (1984) 'Occupational fatigue and preterm birth', in Chamberlain, G. (ed.) *Pregnant women at work*. Royal Society of Medicine, London, pp.87-104.

163 Lokey, E.A., Tran, Z.V., Wells, C.L. Myers, B.C. and Tran, A.C. (1991) 'Effects of physical exercise on pregnancy outcomes: a meta-analytic review', *Medicine and Science in Sports and Exercise*. vol 23, no.11, pp.1234-8.

164 Kramer, M. (1993) 'Regular aerobic exercise during pregnancy', in Enkin, M.W., Keirse, M.J.N.C., Renfrew, M.J. and Neilson, J.P. (eds.) *Pregnancy and Childbirth Module*. Review No.07208, Cochrane Database of Systematic Reviews, Cochrane Updates on Disk, Oxford, Update Software.

165 Pletcher, B.A., Williams, M.K., Multivor, R.A., Barth, D., Linder, C. and Rawlingson, K. (1991) 'Intrauterine cytomegalovirus infection presenting as fetal meconium peritonitis', *Obstetrics and Gynecology*. vol 78, no.5, pp.903-4.

166 Humphrey, W., Magoon, M. and O'Shaughnessy, R. (1991) 'Severe non-immune hydrops secondary to parvovirus B-19 infection: spontaneous reversal in utero and survival of a term infant', *Obstetrics Gynecology*. vol 78, no.5, 1991, pp.900-902.

167 Banatvala, J.E. (1985) 'Rubella – continuing problems', *British Journal of Obstetrics and Gynaecology*. vol 92, pp.193-6.

168 Hiemstra, I., Van Bel, F. and Berger, H.M. (1984) 'Can Trichomonas vaginalis cause pneumonia in newborn babies?', *British Medical Journal*. vol 289, pp.355-6.

169 Miller, E., Nicoll, A., Rousseau, S.A., Sequeira, P.J.L., Hambling, M.H., Smithells, R.W. and Holzel, H. (1987) 'Congenital rubella in babies of south Asian women in England and Wales: an excess and its causes', *British Medical Journal*. vol 294, 1987, pp.737-9.

170 Little, J. and Nicoll, A. (1988) 'The epidemiology and service implications of congenital and constitutional anomalies in ethnic minorities in the United Kingdom', *Paediatric and Perinatal Epidemiology*. vol 2, pp.161-84.

171 Foulton, W., Naessens, A., Mahler, T., De Waele, M., De Catte, M. and De Meuter, F. (1990) 'Prenatal diagnosis of congenital toxoplasmosis', *Obstetrics and Gynecology*. vol 76, no.5, pp.769-772.

172 Joynson, D.H.M. and Payne, R. (1988) 'Screening for toxoplasma in pregnancy'. (Letter), *Lancet*, vol ii, pp.795-6.

173 Joss, A.W.L., Skinner, L.J., Chatterton, J.M.W., Chisholm, S.M., Williams, M.D. and Ho-Yen, D.O. (1988) 'Simultaneous serological screening for congenital cytomegalovirus and toxoplasma infection', *Public Health*. vol 102, pp.409-417.

174 Hall, S.H. (1993) 'How common is congenital toxoplasmosis and what are its clinical manifestations?' *Maternal and Child Health*. vol 18, no.7, pp.204-9.

175 Carter, A.O., Gelmon, S.B., Wells, G.A. and Toepell, A.P. (1989) 'The effectiveness of a prenatal education programme for the prevention of congenital toxoplasmosis', *Epidemiology and Infection*. vol 103, pp.539-545.

176 Rooney, C. (1992) 'Antenatal care and maternal health: how effective is it?', *Maternal Health and Safe Motherhood Programme*. World Health Organization, Geneva.

177 Kaminski, M., Breart, G., Buekens, P., Huisjes, H.J. and McIlwaine, G. (eds.) (1986) *Perinatal care delivery systems: description and evaluation in European community countries*. Oxford Medical Publications, Oxford.

178 Reid, M. and Garcia, J. (1989) 'Women's views of care during pregnancy and childbirth', in Chalmers, I. Enkin, M. and Keirse, M.J.N.C. (eds.) *Effective care in pregnancy and childbirth*. Oxford University Press, Oxford.

179 Hall, M., Macintyre, S. and Porter, M. (1985) *Antenatal care assessed.* Aberdeen University Press, Aberdeen.

180 Howie, P.W., McIlwaine, G. and Florey, C. (1991) *What is antenatal care in Scotland?.* Report to the Scottish Home and Health Department.

181 Neilson, J.P. (1993) 'Routine ultrasonography in early pregnancy', in Enkin, M.W., Keirse, M.J.N.C., Renfrew, M.J. and Neilson, J.P. (eds.) *Pregnancy and childbirth module.* Review No. 03872, Cochrane Database of Systematic Reviews Cochrane Updates on Disk, Oxford, Update Software.

182 Medical Research Council (1991) 'Working Party on the evaluation of chorion villus sampling', *Lancet.* vol 337, pp.1491–9.

183 Watson, E. (1984) 'Health of infants and use of health services by mothers of different ethnic groups in East London', *Community Medicine.* vol 6, pp.127–135.

184 Green, J.M. and France-Dawson, M. (1993) 'Women's experiences of routine screening during pregnancy: the sickle cell study', in *Targeting health promotion: reaching those in need - proceedings of a symposium.* Health Promotion Research Trust, Cambridge, vol 4, no.23.

185 Pheonix, A. (1990) 'Black women and the maternity services', in Garcia, J., Kilpatrick, R. and Richards, M. (eds.) *The politics of maternity care.* Oxford. Clarendon Press, Oxford.

186 National Association of Health Authorities (1988). *Action not words - a strategy to improve health services for black and minority ethnic groups.* Health Management Information Services, Leeds.

187 Cornwell, J. and Gordon, P. (eds.) (1984) *An Experiment in advocacy - the Hackney Multi Ethnic Women's Health Project.* King's Fund Centre, London.

188 Perfrement, S. (1982) *Women's information on pregnancy, childbirth and babycare.* Centre for Medical Research, University of Sussex, Hove.

189 Chisholm, D.K. (1989) 'Factors associated with late booking for antenatal care in Manchester', *Public Health.* vol 103, pp.459–66.

190 Grimsley, M. and Bhat, A. (1988) 'Health', in Bhat, A. and Carr-Hill, R. (eds.) *Britain's black population.* Gower, Aldershot.

191 Feder, G. and Hussey, R. (1990) 'Traveller mothers and babies', *British Medical Journal.* vol 300, pp.1536–37.

192 Durward, L. (1990) *Traveller mothers and babies: who cares for their health?* Maternity Alliance, London.

193 Watson, C. (1984) 'The vital link', *Nursing Times.* July 25 pp.18–19.

194 Mohammed, S. (1991) 'Improving health services for black populations', *Health and race - creating social change.* Issue 1, November.

195 Parsons, L. and Day, S. (1992) 'Improving obstetric outcomes in ethnic minorities: an evaluation of health advocacy', *Public Health Medicine,* vol 14, no.2, pp.183–191.

196 Department of Health and Social Security (1987) *Asian Mother and Baby Campaign: a report by the Director.* DHSS, London.

197 Rocheron, Y., Dickinson, R. and Khan, S. (1989) *Evaluation of the Asian Mother and Baby Campaign.* University of Leicester: Centre for Mass Communication Research.

198 Rocheron, Y. (1988) 'The Asian Mother and Baby Campaign: the reconstruction of ethnic minorities' health needs', *Critical Social Policy.* vol 22, no.4, p.23.

199 Rocheron, Y. and Dickinson, R. (1990) 'The Asian Mother and Baby Campaign; a way forward in health promotion for Asian women?', *Health Education Journal.* vol 49, no.3, pp.128–33.

200 Mason, E.S. (1990) 'The Asian Mother and Baby Campaign: the Leicestershire experience', *Journal of the Royal Society for Health.* vol 110, pp.1–9.

201 Garcia, J. (1989) *Getting consumers' views of maternity care: examples of how the OPCS Survey Manual can help.* Department of Health, London.

202 Cuckle, H.S. and Wald, N.J. (1984) 'Principles of screening', in Wald, N.J. (ed.) *Antenatal and neonatal screening.* Oxford University Press, Oxford, pp.1–22.

203 Sokal, D.C., Bryd, J.R., Chen, A.T.L., Goldberg, M.F. and Oakley, G.P. Jr. (1980) 'Prenatal chromosomal diagnosis: racial and geographic variation for older women in Georgia', *Journal of the American Medical Association.* vol 244, pp.1355–7.

204 Cavalli-Sforza, L.L. and Bodmer, W.F. (1976) *The genetics of human populations*. Freeman and Co., San Francisco.

205 Royal College of Physicians (1989) *Prenatal diagnosis and genetic screening: community and service implications*. RCP, London.

206 Hoffman, E.P., Brown, R.H. and Kunkel, L.M.(1987) 'Dystrophin: the protein product of the Duchenne muscular dystrophy locus', *Cell*. vol 51, pp.919–28.

207 Modell, B. and Kuliev, A.M. (1992) *Social and genetic implications of customary consanguineous marriage among British Pakistanis*. Report of a meeting held at the Ciba Foundation on 15.1.1991, The Galton Institute.

208 Bundey, S., Alam, H., Kaur, A., Mir, S. and Lancashire, R. (1991) 'Why do UK-born Pakistani babies have high perinatal and neonatal mortality rates?', *Paediatric and Perinatal Epidemiology*. vol 5, pp.101–14.

209 Bittles, A.H. and Makov, E. (1988) 'Inbreeding in human populations: an assessment of costs', In Mascie Taylor, C.G.N. and Boyce, A.J. (eds.) *Human mating patterns*. Cambridge University Press, Cambridge.

210 Campbell, A.V. (1984) 'Ethical issues in prenatal diagnosis', *British Medical Journal*. vol 288, pp.1633–4.

211 Farrant, W. (1980) 'Importance of counselling in antenatal screening', *Mimms Magazine*. pp.63–65.

212 France-Dawson, M. (1990) *Sickle cell conditions – the continuing need for comprehensive health care services: a study of patients' views*. Unit Report, Daphne Heald Research Unit, London.

213 Marteau, T. (1991) 'Psychological implications of prenatal diagnosis', in Drife, J.O. and Donnai, D. (eds.) *Antenatal diagnosis of fetal abnormalities*. Springer-Verlag, London, pp.243–54.

214 Green, J.M. (1990) 'Calming or harming: a critical review of psychological effects of fetal diagnosis on pregnant women', *Galton Institute, Occasional Papers*, Second Series, no. 2.

215 Green, J.M., Snowdon, C. and Statham, H. (1993) 'Pregnant women's attitudes to abortion and prenatal screening', *Journal of Reproductive and Infant Psychology*. vol 11, no.1, pp.31–9.

216 Evers-Kiebooms, G., Denayer, L., Decruyanaere, M. and van den Berge, H. (1993) 'Community attitudes towards prenatal testing for congenital handicap', *Journal of Reproductive and Infant Psychology*. vol 11, no.1, pp.21–30.

217 Marteau, (1991) T.M. 'Psychological implications of prenatal diagnosis' in Drife, J.O. and Donnai, D. (eds.) *Antenatal diagnosis of fetal abnormalities*. Springer-Verlag, London.

218 Sanden, M.-L., and Bjurulf, P. (1988) 'Pregnant women's attitudes for accepting or declining a serum-alpha-fetoprotein test', *Scandinavian Journal of Social Medicine*. vol 16, pp.265–71.

219 Green, J.M., Statham, H. and Snowdon, C. (1993) 'Women's knowledge of prenatal screening tests. 1: Relationships with hospital screening policy and demographic factors', *Journal of Reproductive and Infant Psychology*. vol 11, no.1, pp.11–20.

220 Marteau, T.M., Slack, J., Kidd, J. and Shaw, R.W. (1992) 'Presenting a routine screening test in antenatal care: practice observed', *Public Health*. vol 106, pp.131–41.

221 Department of Health (1993) *Population needs and genetic services: an outline guide*. Department of Health, London.

222 Cox, A.D., Pound, A., Mills, M., Puckering, C. and Owen, A.L. (1991) 'Evaluation of a home visiting and befriending scheme for young mothers: NEWPIN', *Journal of Royal Society of Medicine*. vol 84, pp.217–220.

223 Johnson, Z., Howell, F. and Molloy, B. (1993) 'Community mothers' programme: randomised controlled trial of non-professional intervention in parenting', *British Medical Journal*. vol 306, pp.1449–52.

224 Rowe, J. and Mahoney, P. (1994) *Parent education: Guidance for purchasers and providers*. HEA, London.

225 Inch, S. (1989) 'Antenatal preparation for breastfeeding', in Chalmers, I., Enkin, M. and Keirse, M.J.N.C. (eds.) *Effective care in pregnancy and childbirth*. Oxford University Press, Oxford, pp.335–42.

226 Royal College of Midwives (1991) *Successful breastfeeding*. Churchill Livingstone, London.

227 Akre, J. (ed.) (1989) 'Infant Feeding: the physiological basis', *Bulletin of the World Health Organization*, Suppl. vol 67.

228 Minchin, M.K. (1985) *Breastfeeding matters.* Allen and Unwin, Melbourne.

229 Thompson, M. and Westreich, R. (1989) 'Restriction of mother–infant contact in the immediate postnatal period', in Chalmers, I., Enkin, M. and Keirse, M.J.N.C. (eds.) *Effective care in pregnancy and childbirth.* Oxford University Press, Oxford, pp.1322-30.

230 Romito, P. (1989) 'Unhappiness after childbirth', in Chalmers, I., Enkin, M., Keirse, M. (eds.) *Effective care in pregnancy and childbirth.* Oxford University Press, Oxford.

231 Murphy-Black, T. (1989) *Postnatal care at home: a descriptive study of mothers' needs and the maternity services.* Nursing Research Unit, Edinburgh.

232 Renfrew, M.J. (1989) *Restricted breastfeeding.* Oxford Database of Perinatal Trials, 27 June.

233 Renfrew, M.J. (1989) *Combined oestrogen/ progesterone contraceptive in breastfeeding mothers.* Oxford Database of Perinatal Trials, 5 July.

234 Renfrew, M.J. (1991) *Antenatal breastfeeding education*, in Chalmers, I. (ed.) Oxford Database of Perinatal Trials, Version 1.2. Disk Issue 6, Autumn.

235 Beske, E.J., and Garvis, M.S. (1982) 'Important factors in breastfeeding success', *Maternal and Child Nursing.* vol 7, pp.174-9.

236 Kaplowitz, D.D. and Olson, C.M. (1983) 'The effect of an education program on the decision to breastfeed', *Journal of Nutrition Education.* vol 15, pp.61-5.

237 Wiles, L.S. (1984) 'The effect of prenatal breastfeeding education on breastfeeding success and maternal perception of the infant', *Journal of Obstetric, Gynecologic and Neonatal Nursing.* vol 13, pp.253-7.

238 Grossman, L.K., Harter, C. and Kay, A. (1988) 'Prenatal interventions increase breastfeeding among low income women', *American Journal of Diseases of Childhood.* vol 142, p.404.

239 Jones, D.A. and West, R.R. (1985) 'Lactation nurse increases duration of breastfeeding', *Archives of Disease in Children.* vol 60, pp.772-4.

240 Grossman, L.K., Harter, C. and Kay, A. (1986) 'Postpartum lactation counseling for low-income women', *American Journal of Diseases of Childhood.* vol 141, p.375.

241 Lynch, S.A., Koch, A.M., Hislop, T.G. and Coldman, A.J. (1986) 'Evaluating the effect of a breastfeeding consultant on the duration of breastfeeding', *Canadian Journal of Public Health.* vol 77, pp.190-5.

242 Frank, D.A., Wirtz, S.J., Sorenson, J.R. and Heeren, T. (1987) 'Commercial discharge packs and breastfeeding counseling: effects on infant-feeding practices in a randomised trial', *Pediatrics.* vol 80, no.6, pp.845-54.

243 Bergevin, Y., Dougherty, C. and Kramer, M.S. (1983) 'Do infant formula samples shorten the duration of breastfeeding?', *Lancet.* vol 1, pp.1148-51.

244 Feinstein, J.M., Berkelhamer, J.E., Gruszka, M.E., Wong, C.A. and Carey, A.E. (1986) 'Factors related to early termination of breastfeeding in an urban population', *Pediatrics.* vol 78, pp.210-15.

245 Evans, C.J., Lyons, N.B. and Killien, M.G. (1986) 'The effect of formula samples on breastfeeding practices', *Journal of Obstetrics, Gynecology and Neonatal Nursing.* vol 15, pp.401-5.

246 Renfrew, M.J. (1991) *Provision of free samples to breastfeeding mothers*, in Chalmers, I. (ed.) Oxford Database of Perinatal Trials, Version 1.2, Disk Issue 6, Autumn.

247 Dungy, C.I., Christensen-Szalanski, J., Losch, M. and Russell, D. (1992) 'Effect of discharge samples on duration of breastfeeding'. *Pediatrics.* vol 90, no.2, pp.233-7.

248 Salariya, E.N., Easton, P.M. and Cater, J.I. (1978) 'Duration of breastfeeding after early initiation and frequent feeding', *Lancet.* vol 2, pp. 1141-3.

249 Woolridge, M.W. (1986) 'The anatomy of infant suckling', *Midwifery.* vol 2, pp.164-71.

250 Nicholson, W. (1985) 'Cracked nipples in breastfeeding mothers: a randomised controlled trial of three methods of management', *Nursing Mothers of Australia Newsletter.* vol 21, pp.7-10.

251 Righard, L. and Alade, M.O. (1992) 'Sucking technique and its effect on success of breastfeeding', *Birth*, vol 19, pp.185-9.

252 Garforth, S. and Garcia, J. (1989) 'Breast-feeding policies in Practice – "No wonder they get confused"', *Midwifery*. vol 5, 1989, pp.75–83.

253 Beeken, S. and Waterson, T. (1992) 'Health service support of breastfeeding – are we practising what we preach?', *British Medical Journal*. vol 305, pp.285–7.

254 Riordan, F.A.I. and Thomson, A.P.J. (1993) 'Early presentation of meningococcal disease after media publicity', *Archives of Disease in Childhood*. vol 69, p.711.

255 Boyle, G. and Gillam, S. (1993) 'Parents' views of child health surveillance', *Health Education Journal*. vol 52, pp.42–4

256 McIntosh, J. (1993) 'The perceptions and use of child health clinics in a sample of working class families', *Child Care, Health and Development*. vol 18, pp.133–50.

257 Letter to Health Professionals from CMO, Dr Kenneth Calman, 3 Feb 1994.

258 Peckham, C. et al. (1989) *National Immunisation Study: factors influencing immunisation uptake in children*. Action Research for the Crippled Child, London.

259 Holden, J.M., Sagovsky, R. and Cox, J.L. (1989) 'Counselling in a general practice setting: a controlled study of health visitor intervention in treatment of postnatal depression', *British Medical Journal*. vol 298, 1989, pp.223–6.

260 Romanus, V., Jonsell, R. and Berquist, S.O. (1987) 'Pertussis in Sweden after the cessation of general immunisation in 1979', *Paediatric Infectious Disease*. vol 6, pp.364–371.

261 *Health and Personal Social Services Statistics for England* (1993) HMSO, London.

262 Communicable Disease Report: Cover, Vol 4, No 2 – CDSC/PHLS; 4 Feb 1994.

263 HEA/BMRB *Communications Monitor 1993*. London: HEA, 1993.

264 Bennett, P. and Smith, S. (1992) 'Parents' attitudinal and social influences on childhood vaccination', *Health Education Research*. vol 7, no.3, pp.341–8.

265 Barlow, H. and Walker, D. (1990) 'Immunisation in Fife Part II – failure to immunise against whooping cough – reasons given by parents', *Health Education Journal*. vol 49, no.3, pp.103–5.

266 Pearson, M., Makowiecka, M., Gregg, J., Woolard, J., Rogers, M. and West, C. (1993) 'Primary immunisations in Liverpool, I: Who withholds consent?' *Archives of Disease in Childhood*, vol 69, pp.110–14.

267 Hewitt, M. (1989) 'Incidence of contra-indications to immunisation', *Archives of Diseases in Childhood*. vol 64, pp.1052–64.

268 Rogers and Pilgrim. (1993) *Rational non-compliance with childhood immunisation: personal accounts of parents and professionals*. HEA, London.

269 Department of Health (1993) *Report of the Chief Medical Officers Expert Group on the sleeping position of infants and cot death*. Press release H93/786.

270 Downing, C. and Franklin, J. (1989) 'An evaluation of two local infant restraint loan schemes', *First World Conference on Accident and Injury Prevention: Secondary Conference on Child Accident Prevention*. Stockholm.

271 Gray, J.D., Cutler, C.A., Dean, J.G. and Kempe, C.H. (1977) 'Prediction and prevention of child abuse and neglect', *Child Abuse and Neglect International Journal*. vol 1, pp.45–56.

272 Siegel, E., Bauman, K.E., Schaefer, E.S., Saunders, M.M. and Ingram, D.D. (1980) 'Hospital and home support during infancy: impact on maternal attachment, child abuse and neglect, and health care utilisation', *Pediatrics*. vol 66, no.2, pp.183–90.